T0208030

Health Education
for Young Adults

Health Education for Young Adults

A Community Outreach Program

Fabrizia Faustinella, M.D., Ph.D.

Raye Hurwitz, M.D., M.P.H.

Rev. date: 12/13/2018

To order additional copies of this book, contact:
Xlibris
1-888-795-4274
www.Xlibris.com
Orders@Xlibris.com
767844

Contents

Part II

Introduction

Growing up involves changes in your body, the drive to challenge limits and the desire to be part of a group; so why should you bother with a book about your health? So many problems later in life are caused by doing or by not doing something many years before. Why should you bother with that now? We want to give you some good reasons.

To be independent you need to be responsible for yourself. In terms of your health, that means taking care of yourself. Taking care of yourself means taking care of your body and your mind. We often talk about a person's brain and the rest of the body as if they were separate, but in fact, these are part of the same whole, and what you do in terms of your diet, physical activity and rest, as well as potential drug use, smoking and consumption of alcohol, affects the whole person.

As you move into the adolescent years and your body type becomes more adult, your dietary requirements will also change. In our society we often eat food for reasons that have nothing to do with nutrition. We get mixed messages about food. Food is often equated with love, fun and pleasure, yet our culture focuses on the attractiveness of being thin as a goal in itself. We are bombarded by commercials advertising food, as the goal of the food manufacturing industry and the goal of the diet industry is the same, which is to sell more of their products. That's why knowing what a healthy, balanced diet is about is so critical since younger age.

Data from the National Health and Nutrition Examination Survey (NHANES, www.cdc.gov), a program of studies designed to assess the health and nutritional status of adults and children in the United States, revealed that very large numbers of children and teenagers already have poor health behaviors and risk factors for coronary artery disease. Even though coronary artery disease develops between middle and old age, poor health habits in adolescents must be addressed very aggressively to alter the disease prevalence later in life. Coronary artery disease in adults is, at least in part, the outcome of poor health behavior that begins during youth. Many teenagers have at least one predisposing risk factor for heart disease such as obesity, physical inactivity, high cholesterol, hypertension or cigarette smoking. These findings are alarming and show that much needs to be done earlier in life to prevent coronary artery disease later in adulthood.

We know that soldiers who died in the Viet Nam War were found at autopsy to have cholesterol plaques in the arteries of their heart. Many of these young men were only a few years older than you are and their bodies already showed the effects of eating a high fat diet.

It is all right to have occasional snacks if you don't overeat or skip regular meals and if the snacks are nutritious. Many foods have nutritional value in moderation but may not be so good for you in large amounts. Ice cream, for example, can provide calcium, protein and other valuable nutrients, but, in excess, the calories from sugar and fat may become a problem. Chips may provide energy from carbohydrates, but they are usually high in salt, which may contribute to high blood pressure, and in fat. Many people have problems eating the right amount and the right kinds of food. In this book, we'll discuss how to maintain a healthy weight and a positive body image, avoiding diet gimmicks, eating a well-balanced diet, full of a variety of foods that are low in fat and high in fiber, and exercising regularly. Did you know that people don't eat only because they are hungry? They may eat as a result of feelings of sadness or loneliness or boredom, as if to try to fill up when something else is missing. Concerns about appearance, interaction with peers and mounting societal pressures may cause psychological problems and self-esteem issues. As a result of this, the rate of eating disorders, such as anorexia, bulimia and binge eating, is increasing, and not only in young women and girls but also in boys. The physical and emotional consequences of eating disorders can be quite serious, even fatal, and will be addressed in later chapters.

Do you know that physical exercise is important for your brain as well as your body? Substances called endorphins are released with exercise. Endorphins actually make us feel better with a "natural high". Your body needs to be used to stay fit. Stretching and exercise keep us limber and energetic, and builds strong muscles and bones. Find some activity that you like and that is convenient to your schedule and do it at least three or four times per week. Just as you need activity, you need rest and not just for the body. You need to rest your brain as well so it can function effectively when you wake up. Sleep is the process of resting your brain. Specialists consider nine and one half hours per day of sleep necessary for adolescents because this matches the time for growth hormones release at night. Over time the loss of sleep is cumulative and is referred to as 'sleep debt'. If you miss two hours of sleep each day for five days, you have lost a full night of sleep. Trying to make up for lost sleep is not a successful strategy. Staying up late at night to study or party may disrupt your sleep pattern. Decreased sleep contributes to irritability, frustration, depressed mood and difficulty handling emotions. This may lead to problems coping and interacting with people. Judgment can be diminished as well. Concentration and attention can be affected and may foster problems with schoolwork.

Now, think of a movie star, a famous singer or a model smoking a cigarette. It seems like a cool, glamorous image. Now, think of brown teeth, stale breath, wrinkled skin, and yellow nails. Cool? Glamorous? Is it worth smoking for the promise of brown teeth, stale breath, wrinkled skin, and yellow nails? All this will likely happen to you in addition to increased risk of cancer of the mouth, throat, neck, esophagus, lung, bladder and colon, heart disease and stroke. Not being able to breathe is a real "drag" for people with emphysema. Why would any reasonable person fill their lungs with charcoal when we know how much damage it does?

While later in life, small amounts of red wine may be beneficial in lowering cholesterol, during adolescence, however, the risk from alcoholic beverages far outweighs any benefits. When you are trying to establish your place as part of a group, someone may offer you an alcoholic beverage and suggest that drinking is part of being one of the group. It may seem harmless and fun, but think again. Not only does alcohol contribute to motor vehicle crashes, but also it may cause liver damage, brain damage, and cancer. Alcohol dulls your judgment and slows down your reflexes making you less able to make reasonable decisions and be responsible for yourself, with possible devastating consequences which could affect the rest of your life.

The rejection of drug use in our society is determined by many factors including social mores and danger to your health. Our society certainly values productivity and finds disfavor in addictive behavior. Whether you agree with social rules or not, the fact remains that if a substance is illegal, you assume serious legal risks for using them and need to consider the ramifications. Although drug use may seem exciting and certain groups may encourage it, the reality is that use of illegal substances may lead to health problems, death, as well arrest, prosecution, and incarceration. Alcohol and drugs are also linked to early sexual experimentation, which may cause significant problems in terms of contraction of sexually transmitted diseases and unwanted pregnancies.

In addition to poor diet, sedentary life style, smoking, drug and alcohol use, behaviors that might have a negative effect on your health include tattooing, body piercing, sun exposure and exposure to loud noises. Body decorating is a worldwide phenomenon and is practiced regularly in many societies long before the current rage in the United States and western world. The more permanent design placement of tattoos has gained a wider popularity in the U.S. and in western society during the past decades. Formerly considered part of a trucker, seafarer, motorcycle, or military sub-culture, tattooing has been absorbed into the larger culture. The process of tattooing, however, carries greater risks than do other less permanent forms of painting. Skin penetration with needles and the possibility of improper sterilization between users raises the danger of transferring a viral infection from one client to the next. Hepatitis C and HIV are serious consequences. Other problems include skin allergic reactions to the dyes used in tattooing, with development of dermatitis. Once a tattoo is placed, it may be a challenge to have it removed. The process is expensive and painful.

Body piercing is another decorative process that has been widely present in other cultures long before the current popularity in our society. Piercing the nose is a symbol of beauty among the women in the Indian sub-continent. Piercing the nose or stretching the lips is a tradition in parts of Africa. Ear piercing has been an accepted prerogative of European women for centuries. In the late twentieth century, body piercing extended into less traditional parts of the body, such as the tongue, nipples, umbilicus (belly button), clitoris, and penis. What may have started as the identifying symbol of a small group, then spread into the larger culture; for example, ear piercing was common in gay men and later became popular among straight men. These practices may be a symbol of rebelliousness, of belonging, or of a desire to experiment with the latest fad. Again, however, what is important here from a medical perspective is that body piercing carries several risks. A common problem is a hypersensitivity reaction to the metal stud with resulting inflammation and pain of the affected area. Nickel is one of the most common triggers of this type of allergic reaction. Some people may not be able to tolerate any metal except for gold. More serious complications include bacterial infections of the skin and of the mouth, which require treatment with antibiotics. Spread of HIV infection from oral piercing has been documented in the United States and in Europe. Although piercing studios may claim to use sterile instruments, there is no assurance that adequate safety procedures are being followed. Tongue and lip piercing may lead to other non-life threatening complications such as bad breath, drooling, slurred speech and chipped teeth. All of these complications are the reason why the American Dental Association (www.ada.org) has announced their opposition to oral piercing and has published a pamphlet to inform young people of the hazards associated with this practice.

Skin color preferences may change with the times. Hollywood previously exalted the pale look of its Caucasian starlets, but in more recent times, a tanned body became the fashionable ideal. Tanning may give a healthy appearance, but eventually will result in premature aging of the skin. Sun exposure, besides being the greatest cause of skin cancer, is one of the major factors causing skin wrinkles. This change occurs because the sun's ultraviolet rays damage the tissue in the skin that allows elasticity. Fortunately, there are products available now which provide some protection from sun damage. Sunscreens offer a variety of degrees of reduction in the effect of the harmful rays of the sun. The higher the number of the sunscreen is, the higher the protection is. These products need to be applied carefully to all exposed areas of the body and need to be reapplied if washed or rubbed off. The most successful protection is avoidance. Try to stay out of the sun between 10:00 AM and 3:00 PM when the sun's rays are strongest. It is helpful to wear wide-brimmed hats. Some brands of specially treated clothing are available that resist penetration of the sun's rays more than regular clothing.

Sun exposure, besides causing premature skin aging, is by far the greatest cause of all skin cancer. This is true regardless of whether you tan by sun bathing or by using artificial light. Ultraviolet (UV) radiation from the sun is the number one cause of skin cancer, but UV light from tanning beds is just as harmful. Cumulative sun exposure causes mainly basal cell and squamous cell skin cancer, while episodes of severe sunburns, usually before age 18, can cause melanoma later in life.

It is estimated that nearly 9,500 people in the U.S. are diagnosed with skin cancer every day. Researchers estimate that 5.4 million cases of non-melanoma skin cancer, including basal cell carcinoma and squamous cell carcinoma, were treated in 3.3 million people in the United States in 2012 (American Academy of Dermatology, www.aad.org/media/stats/conditions/skin-cancer)

If a cancer is found early, it can be treated and leave little or no skin changes. Others are far more serious. Basal cell cancer can erode the skin, notably occurring on the face, requiring significant tissue removal and resulting in obvious defects. Malignant melanoma is even more dangerous, because of the propensity for metastasizing (spreading to other parts of the body), and treatment may include chemotherapy. One person dies of melanoma every hour (every 54 minutes). An estimated 87,110 new cases of invasive melanoma will be diagnosed in the U.S. in 2017. An estimated 9,730 people will die of melanoma in 2017. Melanoma accounts for less than one percent of skin cancer cases, but the vast majority of skin cancer deaths.

Excessive sun exposure affects the eyes as well, with increased incidence of cataracts development. The regular use of sunglasses will help you to minimize this problem.

Across age groups, hearing loss can result from a variety of causes. Illnesses, genetics, injuries to the head or ear, birth complications or exposure to certain medications can all be factors. Among older people hearing loss is most often attributed to a natural aging of the auditory nerve, also known as age-related hearing loss. In teens, however the most common cause of hearing loss is excessive noise exposure, which is completely preventable.

According to the Journal of Pediatrics, 12.5 percent of kids between the ages of 6 and 19 have hearing loss as a result of listening to loud music, particularly through ear buds at unsafe volumes. Noise induced hearing loss is a problem that previously affected people employed in industries where there is a high noise level caused by the use of power tools. The era of rock music, however, has added a new dimension to the problem of hearing loss. Loud rock music may certainly cause hearing loss, but it will not be immediately obvious and becomes noticeable ten to fifteen years after repeated exposure. The damage will be sensorineural; it affects the nerves that are involved with hearing. With increasing rates of hearing loss comes academic challenges, a growing problem for young people. Kids and teens with hearing loss are at risk academically. If the hearing loss is left untreated, it can affects everything from education to social life to confidence level and vocational choices. Ask your doctor how to protect your hearing.

All high school students should be prepared to make healthy lifestyle choices by receiving straightforward information about basic anatomy and physiology, heart disease risk factors, diet, exercise, the risks of unprotected and premature sexual experimentation, stress management, substance dependence/abuse, including alcohol, tobacco, and other drugs. When Tom Hanks was asked by a reporter what he would do differently if he could go back in time, he answered, among other things, "I would watch my sugar intake".

Being fully aware of how your behavior and your choices earlier in life can have a detrimental effect on your health, now and later, will give you the tools to develop mature and independent thinking, to prevent a vast array of medical problems and disease processes and will allow you to choose a healthy life style.

While we discourage you from looking up your symptoms and health concerns in Google, in an attempt to make your own diagnoses, as this will inevitably cause unnecessary worries and anxiety, we want you to be aware of the fact that there is a plethora of legitimate, medical and governmental, website with accurate and up-to-date information on pretty much every existing illness and disease process, with detailed explanations of causes, risk factors, prevention and treatment. You can easily access these websites from your computer and even from your cell phone. Many of these websites have been used in this book as references and have been mentioned in the pertinent chapters.

You can definitely take advantage of the internet revolution to boost your knowledge, but keep in mind that the best place to start asking questions is in the doctor's office.

Part I

Primary Care and Prevention

In The Doctor's Office

People living in the United States and other western countries are living much longer lives than people did in the past. There are several explanations for this. One reason is the improvement in environmental conditions including the use of sanitation, water purification, and secure housing. Another reason is the advancement in medical science and the emphasis on preventative care. There are established recommendations for different types of screening and vaccinations and when they should occur from infancy through childhood, adolescence, and adulthood. Doctor's visits will therefore allow you to have a physician review your needs, evaluate your growth and development and address your health concerns, both physical and psychological.

Besides physical illnesses, concerns with appearance, interaction with peers and mounting societal pressures may cause psychological problems that can also be addressed in the doctor's office.

The annual "well care" visits don't involve many laboratory screening tests. Rather, the emphasis is on addressing teen health issues, such as accident and injury prevention, sexual health, and avoiding substance abuse. Preventive medicine for teens should emphasize healthy lifestyle choices that help protect against diseases that occur in adulthood.

The American Academy of Pediatrics (AAP) has developed a set of comprehensive health guidelines for well-child care, called Bright Futures, for pediatricians to follow from birth to age 21 (https://brightfutures.aap.org; https://kidshealth.org/en/parents/medical-care). The general recommendations for adolescents between the ages of thirteen and eighteen include a routine check-up every year during which weight, height, blood pressure, vision and hearing will be checked; the body mass index, BMI, will be calculated; screening will be provided, when indicated, for obesity, eating disorders, depression/risk of suicide, alcohol and drug abuse and sexually transmitted diseases (STDs). Laboratory tests can be requested, at the physician's discretion, to check blood glucose and cholesterol level, hemoglobin level, urine analysis and others, if indicated.

An oral exam during a routine visit should also be performed with a dental referral, if necessary. Teens are also checked for musculoskeletal problems, including joint problems and scoliosis, which is a curvature of the spine, not uncommon in growing adolescents. These problems, in addition to asthma/reactive airway disease and heart conditions, could be aggravated by physical activity. Therefore, the physician will evaluate the adolescent and provide recommendations in order to treat and/or prevent worsening of medical conditions and potentially life-threatening problems during physical exercise. Most of the fatalities that occur in adolescent athletes are due to sudden cardiac death, which is caused by underlying congenital (existing from birth) abnormalities of the heart. These include problems with the heart valves, the heart muscle itself, or with the rhythm of the heart and will be discussed in more details in a later chapter.

During puberty, issues related to sexual health will be addressed. Young women may need to be referred for a first visit with a gynecologist; young men should be checked for hernias and testicular cancer and taught how to do a testicular self-exam. While women are generally aware of the magnitude and implication of breast cancer, many young men are unaware of the need to perform self-examinations for evidence of testicular cancer. Women are encouraged to begin breast self-examination in the twenties when, unfortunately, breast cancer may occur, although it is certainly more common later in life. Young men should also perform a testicular self-examination since testicular cancer affects men between the ages of fifteen and forty. It is very easy for a young man to begin a habit of testicular self-examination every month in order to discover any changes in the testicular glands at an early stage and offer a better chance at treatment.

In the doctor's office, adolescents should also receive information and counseling about risky behaviors and other issues, including:
- sexual activities that may result in unintended pregnancy and STDs
- use of alcohol and other substances, including anabolic steroids
- use of tobacco products, including cigarettes and smokeless tobacco
- drinking and driving
- texting and driving
- the importance of bicycle helmets, seatbelts, and protective sports gear

- how to resolve conflicts without violence, including how to avoid the use of weapons
- learning problems or difficulties at school
- importance of regular physical activity
- emotional/behavioral issues

This is a time when you can discuss with your doctor concerns about your weight or height, problems with family and friends, difficulties in school, and sexual issues or assault. The doctor may help you understand the danger of alcohol, tobacco, steroids, and other drug use, and help you quit. Remember that sports authorities and prospective employers may perform drug screens for eligibility. This may even include nicotine.

Finally, don't forget about vaccinations.
The following immunizations should be received by age 13:
- chickenpox (varicella) vaccine (if they have not had chickenpox)
- measles, mumps, and rubella (MMR) vaccine
- hepatitis B vaccine (HBV) series
- hepatitis A vaccine (HAV) series
- meningococcal vaccine
- human papillomavirus vaccine (HPV)
- diphtheria, tetanus, and acellular pertussis booster (Tdap)

Doctors recommend a Tdap booster at 11–12 years of age, with a tetanus and diphtheria booster (Td) every 10 years after that. The Tdap vaccine is also recommended for all pregnant women during the second half of each pregnancy, regardless of whether or not they had it before, or when it was last given. The flu vaccine, given before flu season each year, also is recommended.

Adolescents at high risk for pneumococcal diseases such as those with Sickle Cell Disease or other immunosuppressed states should receive the pneumococcal vaccine. Colleges and universities now require up to date vaccination in order to be enrolled in their institution.

Three vaccines (Cevarix, Gardasil, Gardasil-9) are now available to protect against cancer of the cervix, penis, mouth, or throat, which might be caused by HPV (Human Papilloma Virus). Gardasil and Gardasil-9 also protect against genital warts, vaginal cancer, and anal cancer. The CDC recommends young women ages 11 to 26 and young men ages 11 to 21 get vaccinated for HPV.

Today's generation of children and adolescents is growing up immersed in media. This includes platforms that allow users to both consume and create content, social and interactive media that can be creative and engaging, sedentary and active video games and highly immersive virtual reality. Parents play an important role in helping children and teens navigate media, which can have both positive and negative effects. For school-aged children and adolescents, the idea is to balance media use with other healthy behaviors. Problems start when media use displaces physical activity, hands-on exploration and face-to-face social interaction in the real world, which is critical to learning. Too much screen time can also harm the amount and quality of sleep. In this context, counseling at the physician's office is yet another opportunity to discuss choices for a healthy life style.

www.cdc.gov
www.ada.org
www.aad.org/media/stats/conditions/skin-cancer
https://brightfutures.aap.org
www.uspreventiveservicestaskforce.org

www.mentalhealth.gov
https://kidshealth.org/en/parents/medical-care

Leading Causes of Death and Prevention

Life expectancy has reached a record high of 78.8 years, for all races and origins in the United States, as shown in the 2012 National Vitals Statistics Report (www.cdc.gov). How likely do you think you are to live so long? Let us first look at the leading causes of death in the United States for people ages thirteen through nineteen.

Deaths to teenagers 12–19 years is a small fraction of the total deaths occurring each year in the United States. From 1999 to 2006 less than 1 percent (0.68 percent), or 131,000 deaths, occurred to teenagers 12–19 years. This represents an average of 16,375 deaths per year for this group.

Teenage mortality is an important public health issue because the majority of deaths among teenagers are caused by external causes of injury such as accidents, homicide and suicide. These causes of death are therefore preventable.

The Centers For Disease Control and Prevention (CDC) estimates that each year from 1999 to 2006, the annual death rate for teenagers has averaged 49.5 deaths per 100,000 population. However, the risk of dying is not distributed evenly among all teenagers. Male teenagers are more likely to die than female teenagers at every single year of age from 12 to 19 years, and older teenagers are at higher risk of dying than younger teenagers. At age 12, for example, the death rate for males is 46 percent higher than the rate for females. At age 19 the death rate for males is almost three times the rate for females.

Among teenagers 12–19 years, death rates increase with every additional year of age. This pattern is stronger for males. Starting at age 12 and ending at 19 years, the death rate among teenage males increases 32 percent on average for every additional year of age. For females, on the other hand, the death rate increases on average 19.5 percent for every additional year of age.

What are the leading causes of death for teenagers?

The leading causes of death for the teenage population remained constant throughout the period 1999–2006: Accidents (unintentional injuries) (48 percent of deaths), homicide (13 percent), suicide (11 percent), cancer (6 percent), and heart disease (3 percent). Motor vehicle accident accounted for almost three quarters (73 percent) of all deaths from unintentional injury.

The death rate for teenagers 12–19 years varies by sex, race, and Hispanic origin. Non-Hispanic black teenagers are 37 percent more likely to die than Hispanic and non-Hispanic white teenagers.

The death rate for non-Hispanic black teenagers is 64.5 deaths per 100,000 population compared with 47.1 for Hispanic and 47.0 for non-Hispanic white teenagers. Therefore, the death rate for non-Hispanic black male teenagers is the highest, at 94.1 deaths per 100,000 population.

Non-Hispanic black male teenagers are disproportionately affected by homicide. While homicide is the second cause of death among adolescents as a group, it is the leading cause of death for non-Hispanic black male teenagers. The risk of dying from homicide among non-Hispanic black male teenagers is more than twice that of Hispanic males and about 15 times that of non-Hispanic white males.

How can we modify behaviors in order to reduce the primary causes of death in adolescents?

As it relates to motor vehicle crashes, we can strongly recommend using seat belts, restricting the number of passengers, and not driving under the influence of alcohol or other drugs. Alcohol is frequently involved in adolescent driver fatalities. Alcohol is also involved in adolescent drowning. Besides being a primary cause of death, motor vehicle crashes can result in permanent damage such as traumatic head injury, paralysis or limb amputation and disfiguration, affecting your life dramatically. Adolescents should be reminded that bicycles and motorcycles are vehicles as well, and riders must obey traffic laws, just as automobile drivers must. Riders should also wear a helmet, as many severe bicycle-related injuries and deaths could have been prevented by wearing one.

Homicide is the second leading cause of death among adolescents. Unfortunately, we live in a violent society; however, one of the risks of firearm fatalities is actually "playing with a gun". The person who pulls the trigger may be a friend, a family member, or the victim. These causes of death are preventable as well and much needs to be done in the area of gun access and safety.

The third leading cause of death of adolescents is suicide. Suicide affects young people from all races and socioeconomic groups. There has been a dramatic increase in the number of adolescent suicides. Many "accidental" deaths are actually believed to be suicides. It appears that most adolescents who commit suicide have never received mental health treatment, although a majority has exhibited psychiatric symptoms. Obviously, this raises the need for suicide awareness.

Adolescent may attempt suicide by overdosing on prescription drugs such as sleeping pills or on over-the-counter medications, such as Tylenol (acetaminophen) and aspirin (acetyl-salicylic-acid). The intentional overdosing is often a desperate cry for help. The consequences of this action may not be recognized as being life-threatening. Although Tylenol (acetaminophen) and aspirin may be bought without prescription, these drugs are far from harmless in large doses. Overdoses of acetaminophen cause acute liver failure which can be fatal if not treated promptly in an emergency center. Ingesting large quantities of aspirin causes salicylate poisoning which can produce nausea, vomiting, and dangerous disregulation in bodily functions, such as respiration, temperature control, and metabolism. Drugs such a sleeping pills, anti-depressants, cardiac and pain medication that may have been prescribed to a family member may be accessible to a troubled youth. When used inappropriately, these drugs have toxic effects. They may cause life-threatening heart rhythm abnormalities, respiratory failure, coma, and damage to other vital organs.

Adolescent attempt suicide also by using weapons or by hanging. There appears to be an increase in the use of firearms by even the younger teen-age boys. Guns and rifles may be available in the household because of intended self-protection, hunting, or other sporting activities. Whether firearms are registered or owned illegally, their inherent capacity for killing makes them a dangerous tool in the hands of a troubled or inexperienced youth.

Reasons for attempting suicide vary. There may be an underlying treated or undiagnosed psychiatric condition such as depression or bipolar disorder or a family history of suicide that increase the risk of suicide. As mentioned above, most adolescents who commit suicide have never received mental health treatment, although many have exhibited psychiatric symptoms. Use of alcohol and drugs are associated with suicidal behavior. They cause impaired judgment resulting in mood disturbances such as depression, or cognitive disturbances such as psychosis.

Another social behavior that affects morbidity and mortality in adolescents is abusive relationships. Unfortunately, many children and adolescents are exposed to less than loving family environments. They may be harmed by someone who is considered a friend of the family but who takes advantage of them. They may even be abused by their parents who may be under the influence of alcohol or other drugs or be otherwise unable to provide a healthy environment for their children. The parents may feel increasingly stressed from the pressures of their own lives and may react against their own families. Domestic violence may be physical or psychological. Victims of abuse may develop depression and anxiety. They may develop physical symptoms such as headache, stomachache or generalized aches and pains. Drug abuse and suicide attempts may be tragic outcomes of domestic violence. Teenagers may also find themselves in relationships with their peers that are destructive. While a certain amount of conflict is a normal part of interaction, bullying is a dangerous threat to teenage well-being and social development. Bullying is a specific type of aggression in which the behavior is intended to harm or disturb the other person, the behavior occurs repetitively over time, and there is an imbalance of power with a more powerful person or group attacking a less powerful one. The aggressive behavior may be verbal (name-calling and threats), physical assault (beating, pushing or shoving), or psychological (intimidation and isolation). Both the youth who bully others and those who are bullied are at high risk for aggressive behavior.

Both groups demonstrate problems with social and emotional adjustment. Teens who are bullied may feel loss of self-esteem. There have been recent instances in which teens who were the objects of continued bullying or intolerance have reacted violently, towards themselves or others, with catastrophic consequences. It should not be taken lightly if a boy or a girl is emotionally or physically abusive with his/her supposed friend or acquaintance. This type of activity takes on group sanction when it is part of sorority/fraternity hazing and has, unfortunately, achieved acceptance in parts of our society. Having one's friend die from a tragic incident under the pretense of becoming part of a group/gang makes this type of activity clearly one of violence rather than sport or camaraderie.

The adolescent who is physically and sexually abused may be pushed towards thoughts of suicide as a result of a sense of hopelessness. Older children and teenagers may spend time after school and on weekends unsupervised and without meaningful social connections. Their parents may be unavailable to them due to work demands or to their own emotional needs. This can lead to a young person's sense of isolation. Teenagers may also be profoundly affected by their peer's exclusion of them from social activities. Their sense of rejection may have tragic consequences, as we have seen in the terrible instances of mass killings. All this raises the need for suicide awareness among adolescents.

Your awareness and your keen insights are extraordinarily important. If you experience a sense of profound sadness or feel at a loss as to how to cope or if you notice behavior in a friend or acquaintance that makes you uncomfortable, find an adult in whom to confide. There are people available to you. Certainly, your parents are your first source for help and advice. If they are unavailable for whatever reason, look to a favorite relative, school teacher, counselor, coach, or physician, for assistance with your own pain or to intervene to help a friend in pain.

Fitness

Fitness refers to good physical condition resulting from exercise and proper nutrition. Fitness includes both a physical and an emotional component. Both components require preparation and certain skills that may improve with training. Some specialized forms of physical activity, such as yoga, incorporate a focus on mental aspects as well, and exemplify the "mind-body" concept that has gained much popularity in our society.

There is some inevitable loss of muscle strength as we age; those who exercise regularly, however, are likely to be more fit than their sedentary contemporaries and possibly more fit than much younger people who are inactive. The medical characteristics that are associated with aging overlap those associated with inactivity and include a decrease in cardiovascular function, muscle mass, strength, flexibility, and bone mass, as well as an increase in body fat and sleep disturbances.

The 2008 Physical Activity Guidelines for Americans issued by the US Department of Health and Human Services, recommend that children and adolescents aged 6 to 17 years should have 60 minutes or more of physical activity each day. Most of the 60 or more minutes a day should be either moderate- or vigorous-intensity aerobic physical activity and should include vigorous-intensity physical activity at least 3 days a week.

As part of their 60 or more minutes of daily physical activity, children and adolescents should include muscle-strengthening physical activity and bone-strengthening physical activity on at least 3 days of the week.

Physical activity may be divided into two types: aerobic and anaerobic exercise. Anaerobic exercise, such as weight-lifting or pushups, involves short bursts of activity which build muscle, strength and mass. It offers little benefit for cardiovascular conditioning. Aerobic exercise, such as brisk walking, swimming, or biking, involves moderate activity for a sustained period of time and improves both cardiovascular and muscular efficiency. Most team sports involve a combination of the two. Cross-training, being involved in a variety of sports and activities, decreases the risk of injury from overuse of selected muscle groups and contributes to total fitness by involving more muscle groups. An important aspect of exercise is the process of warming up by gradual stretching which contributes in the long term to flexibility and in the short term to joint protection. It is important to find something that you enjoy so that you stick with it.

It is best to have supervision for physical activity that is new or more strenuous for you in order to avoid injury and avoid pushing your cardiovascular function beyond your current level of training. Certain sports have increased risks for immediate injuries or for later problems with osteoarthritis, a degenerative joint condition that damages the cartilage and causes pain and decreased mobility. Activities that increase the risk for osteoarthritis include those that require abrupt and direct impact on a joint as the result of contact with other players or with playing surfaces. Injuries to the knees, shoulders, back and neck are common examples of this in football. Injuries to the knees are common in soccer. Repetitive joint impact also contributes to joint damage in the elbows of baseball pitchers and tennis players and in the knees of soccer players and runners. Attempts should be made to reduce these risks by careful individual evaluation and proper training to improve joint stability. Equipment such as shoulder pads, knee pads and braces may help reduce direct joint impact. Prompt treatment of injuries and appropriate and complete rehabilitation will also decrease the risk of permanent damage.

Back pain is a common problem that develops not only as a result of injuries but also as a result of decreased physical activity and unbalanced use of the different muscle groups. Posture is an important part of this, not just because we are told slouching looks bad. Proper conditioning and use of upper back and abdominal muscles are key to the prevention of many neck and back complaints that develop as people age. Over time, we have a tendency to rely on some muscle groups to the exclusion of others, which results in poor posture and back strain. Strengthening the muscles around the shoulder blades and the abdominal muscles is key to maintaining the back properly aligned and pain-free.

Moderate–intensity aerobic exercise includes:
- Active recreation, such as canoeing, hiking, cross-country skiing, skateboarding, rollerblading
- Brisk walking
- Bicycle riding (stationary or road bike)
- House and yard work such as sweeping or pushing a lawn mower
- Playing games that require catching and throwing, such as baseball, softball, basketball and volleyball

Vigorous –intensity aerobic exercise includes:
- Active games involving running and chasing, such as flag football, soccer
- Bicycle riding

- Jumping rope
- Martial arts such as karate
- Running
- Sports such as tennis, ice or field hockey, basketball, swimming
- Vigorous dancing
- Aerobics
- Cheerleading or gymnastics

Examples of muscle strengthening exercises are:
- Games such as tug of war
- Push-ups
- Resistance exercises with exercise bands, weight machines, hand-held weights
- Rock climbing
- Sit-ups
- Cheerleading or Gymnastics

Bone-strengthening exercises include:
- Hopping, skipping, jumping
- Jumping rope
- Running
- Sports such as gymnastics, basketball, volleyball, tennis

Exercise offers the possibility of physical activity and mental relaxation simultaneously. Benefits of exercise include release of muscle tension, muscle strengthening, increased flexibility and balance, and an enhancement of the ability to handle daily stress by refocusing one's attention. Science has found chemical connections in the interaction of the mind with the body. Hatha yoga is based on achieving specific body positions while maintaining controlled patterns of breathing. Repetitive stretching and mental focusing in yoga reinforces the ability to achieve a relaxation response. This contributes both to overall fitness and sense of wellbeing. The breathing technique used in yoga emphasizes the use of the diaphragm, the muscle that separates the thorax (chest cavity) from the abdomen. This allows a fuller expansion of the lower part of the lungs and increases respiratory efficiency. It also stimulates a relaxation response that contributes to stress reduction. Diaphragmatic breathing is now being applied to more traditional forms of exercise and also to daily life.

Despite the many health benefits associated with regular physical activity, many children and adolescents do not participate in physical activity for 60 minutes or more each day. To promote the guidelines and support youth physical activity, CDC (www.cdc.gov) and several partner organizations developed the Youth Physical Activity Guidelines Toolkit (www.cdc.gov/healthyschools/physicalactivity/guidelines.htm), which highlights strategies that schools, families, and communities can use to support youth physical activity.

The toolkit can be used by anyone who promotes youth physical activity, including community leaders; physical education and health education teachers; physical activity coordinators at the school, district, and state levels; and physical activity practitioners working in health or community-based organizations.

Don't use this as an excuse not to work out, but laughter could offer a small help to your fitness plan. Laughing raises your heart rate and caloric expenditure, resulting in about 10-40 calories burned over 15 minutes of laughter according to a study by the International Journal of Obesity. Recent observations suggest that increased respiration and blood flow to the brain occur with laughing. This has generated a new interest in the physiological and psychological benefits of laughter.

Laughing decreases stress hormone levels, triggers the release of endorphins, lowers blood pressure and create a general sense of wellbeing. So smile, laugh, and live a healthier life!

Diet

Nutritional guidelines are important in adolescence since the growth rate at this time is second only to that during infancy. It is important whether you are active or sedentary to eat a variety of foods from the basic food groups. Americans are obsessed with weight loss for medical and cosmetic reasons. Many different diets have been promoted and have gained different degrees of popularity.

The constant barrage of diet and nutrition information that is published can make it difficult for people to grasp the basic principles of good, healthy nutrition. Despite all the myriad of available diet programs, we believe that The American Heart Association (AHA, www.heart.org) dietary guidelines are a sound starting point for most people, regardless of whether they have heart problems or not. The AHA dietary Guidelines for the General Population are focused on "achieving and maintaining a healthy eating pattern that includes foods from each of the major food groups. Eating adequate amounts of essential nutrients, coupled with energy intake in balance with energy expenditure, is essential to maintain health and to prevent or delay the development of cardiovascular disease, stroke, hypertension, and obesity" (http://circ. ahajournals.org/content/102/18/2284).

The nutritional content varies among different foods and that's why it's critical to eat foods from various food groups, such as fruits and vegetables, low-fat dairy products, cereal and grain products, legumes and nuts, fish, poultry, and lean meats.

Olive and other vegetable oils are the preferred types of oil for this diet, rather than animal fat such as butter and lard. Animal foods, especially eggs, some seafood and meats, are rich in cholesterol and saturated fats, which are also found in some plant foods, such as palm and coconut oil, leading to an increase in blood cholesterol levels, which is a risk factor for heart disease.

Diets rich in fruits, vegetables and grain products are associated with a lower risk of developing heart disease, stroke, and hypertension. Foods high in complex carbohydrates/starches (bread, pasta, cereal, potatoes) are definitely recommended over foods rich in sugars/simple carbohydrates. Grains, vegetables, fruits, legumes, and nuts are also good sources of fibers, which may contribute to lower the cholesterol level.

Vitamin and mineral supplements should not be seen as a substitute for a balanced and nutritious diet which emphasizes the intake of fruits, vegetables, and grains. Being mindful of portion number and size is very important as well to avoid excessive calorie intake and adequate nutrition.

Your goal should be to achieve and maintain a healthy body weight, because being overweight is associated with an increased risk of hypertension, diabetes mellitus and cardiovascular disease, later in life.

The body mass index (BMI, in kg/m2) is used to define body composition, with a BMI ≥25.0 and <30.0 defining the overweight state, a BMI ≥30 and <40 defining obesity, and a BMI ≥40 defining extreme obesity. When BMI is excessive (≥25), weight loss should be achieved through healthy diet and exercise programs, with the goal of introducing fewer calories than those burned by physical activity.

Well known diets, which you may have heard about, include the following:

The Atkins diet promotes weight loss by severely limiting carbohydrates, which are the "ready to burn" food source that converts quickly to glucose. Any glucose that is not burned for energy gets stored as fat. By eliminating carbohydrates from the diet, the body naturally breaks down stored fat into chemicals called "ketones" which are burned for energy. Ketones suppress appetite, which also leads to less calorie intake. In the short term, the Atkins diet usually works for weight loss, but there is much controversy over the long-term health effects.

The South-Beach Diet is a "heart-friendly" version similar to the Atkins diet, but it makes a distinction between good and bad carbohydrates, and between good and bad fats. Similar to Atkins, reducing carbs is key, mostly the high-glycemic carbs that so quickly breakdown to glucose. Unlike the Atkins plan, only healthy fats are allowed.

The Pritikin and the Ornish diets are both centered on a low-fat diet. As with the South-Beach diet there is a distinction between good and bad carbs and good and bad fats. The Ornish program in particular emphasizes the diet as part of a bigger program including exercise, stress relief, and healthy social connections. Dr. Ornish has published numerous articles on the success of his program in reversing heart disease, and has succeeded in getting insurances such as Medicare to actually pay for qualifying patients to go through his "intensive cardiac rehabilitation" program.

The Paleo diet, also known as the "caveman" diet, is based on the idea of eating similar to our distant Paleolithic hunter-gatherer ancestors, focusing on a diet that includes wild game, fish, nuts, roots, fruits and vegetables. Excluded are foods that came into our diet after the age of agriculture and domestication of animals – namely grains, legumes, and dairy. Loren Cordain, PhD, Colorado State University professor and author of "The Paleo Diet", says even though grains and dairy seem healthful, our "genome has not really adapted to these foods, which can cause inflammation at the cellular level and promote disease."

The Mediterranean Diet, rich in plant foods and healthy fats, has shown some of the best health benefits of any in numerous studies. The focus is on locally available and fresh seasonal foods, relying heavily on unprocessed, whole plant foods such as fruits and vegetables, beans, whole grains, nuts, olives, and olive oil along with some cheese, yogurt, fish, poultry, eggs, and wine.

The Hormone Diet plan emphasizes the role of hormones in proper metabolism, such as thyroid, cortisol, and the sex hormone, pointing out that balancing hormones is key to good metabolism and weight loss. Promoted by naturopathic doctor Natasha Turner, the plan explains how fluctuations in certain hormone levels may contribute to stubborn belly fat, weight gain, sluggishness, stress, sugar cravings, and health problems.

The plan calls for lifestyle changes, doing a 2-week "detox," and adopting a Mediterranean-style diet that includes certain supplements.

The Zone diet is geared toward eating a balance of foods that lower inflammation and lower insulin levels. Author, Dr. Sears, recommends lower carbohydrate intake and some protein at every meal in order to blunt the fat storage hormone called insulin, and encourage more of the fat breakdown hormone called glucagon. The focus is that we think of food not as "a source of calories but as a control system for hormones."

If you are interested in a vegetarian diet, it is possible to have an adequate diet without eating meat, poultry or fish. It does become more complicated if dairy products (milk, cheese and eggs) are excluded. With these latter foods, however, one is certainly able to obtain an adequate supply of essential proteins and to maintain a healthy diet. It is possible to derive sufficient protein from a diet that excludes meat, poultry, and fish, by eating whole grains, legumes, vegetables, seeds and nuts. Soy protein has been shown to be equal to proteins of animal origin. Non-meat sources can provide most of the critical vitamins and minerals found in meat products, with the exception of B12 that can be found in dairy products and eggs, in some fortified breakfast cereals, fortified soy beverages, as well as vitamin supplements. There are different types of vegetarian diet: the vegan or total vegetarian diet, which includes only foods from plants, such as fruits, vegetables, legumes (dried beans and peas), grains, seeds and nuts; the lactovegetarian diet which includes plant foods and dairy products; the ovo-lactovegetarian (or lacto-ovovegetarian) diet, which, in addition to plant foods and dairy foods, also includes eggs. The semi-vegetarian diet includes chicken and fish with plant foods, dairy products and eggs and excludes red meat.

A vegetarian diet can be healthy, if it's planned to include a broad variety of foods and does have enough calories to meet your energy needs.

Although Americans generally believe that diets excluding meat products are dull, many traditional societies base their diets on a combination of different vegetable sources that lead to what Ms. Lapay calls "protein complementarity", by eating several different types of food, one is more likely to obtain a balance in required nutrients. Doing this also tends to lead to a diet that is higher in fiber and lower in salt, sugar, and fats than the typical American diet which is high in meat and processed food. Fast food or processed food products have hidden but high amounts of salt, fat, and sugar. We have mentioned previously the particular risks of salt in contributing to hypertension, sugar to obesity and diabetes, and fat to cardiovascular disease.

Unfortunately, many adolescents eat unbalanced diets in which fat and sugar furnish a large percentage of their total calories.

Setting guidelines for weight is based on the concept that weight is related to mortality later in life. Obesity is associated with an increased risk of diabetes, hypertension, and heart disease. On the other hand, being too thin can also be hazardous by increasing the risk for osteoporosis. Since many adolescent girls are preoccupied with being excessively thin, they place themselves at risk for nutritional deficiencies. Diets that are well-balanced are generally recommended by doctors and nutritionists. Fad diets are usually excessively restrictive. They may be nutritionally inadequate because of their lack of balance and poor variety. This can result in growth retardation, pubertal delay, and impairment of calcium deposition in the growing bones. Adolescence is the most critical time for building strong bone. A balanced diet will generally assure adequate intake of all vitamins (A, B complex including thiamine, riboflavin, pyridoxine, and cobalamin, biotin, C, D, E, folic acid, K, niacin, and pantothenic acid) and essential minerals (iron, potassium, iodine, calcium, zinc, selenium, and chromium). Therefore, the practice of using mega doses of over-the-counter vitamins and minerals does not offer any significant advantage and is not beneficial to your health. Nevertheless one multi-vitamin per day may be a reasonable option.

Fluid intake is an important aspect of nutritional maintenance and electrolyte balance. About 90% of our body is actually composed of water molecules. We have to replenish fluids constantly since they are lost during normal bodily processes (sweating, breathing, urination). Additional fluid is lost with physical exercise, increases in ambient temperature, febrile illnesses, and diseases causing vomiting and diarrhea. In these circumstances, remember to drink fluids high in electrolytes, rather than simply water. We cannot emphasize enough how important it is to maintain an adequate fluid intake. Unfortunately, many adolescents rely on beverages high in sugar and caffeine, which, actually, lead to additional fluid loss instead of replenishment.

Energy drinks are widely promoted as products that increase alertness and enhance physical and mental performance. Marketing targeted at young people has been quite effective. Next to multivitamins, energy drinks are the most popular dietary supplement consumed by American teens and young adults. Males between the ages of 18 and 34 years consume the most energy drinks, and almost one-third of teens between 12 and 17 years drink them regularly. Many energy drinks contain as much as 25–50 g of simple sugars; this may be problematic for people who are diabetic or prediabetic. In addition to sugars, caffeine is the major ingredient in most energy drinks—a 24-oz energy drink may contain as much as 500 mg of caffeine (similar to that in four or five cups of coffee). The amounts of caffeine in energy drinks vary widely, and the actual caffeine content may not be identified easily. Guarana, commonly added to energy drinks, contains caffeine. Therefore, the addition of guarana increases the drink's total caffeine content. Consuming energy drinks increases important safety concerns. Between 2007 and 2011, the overall number of energy-drink related visits to emergency departments doubled, with the most significant increase (279 percent) in people aged 40 and older. A growing trend among young adults and teens is mixing energy drinks with alcohol. About 25 percent of college students consume alcohol with energy drinks, and they binge-drink significantly more often than students who don't mix them. In 2011, 42 percent of all energy-drink related emergency department visits involved combining these beverages with alcohol or drugs (including illicit drugs, like marijuana, as well as central nervous system stimulants, like Ritalin or Adderall).

Although there's very limited data that caffeine-containing energy drinks may temporarily improve alertness and physical endurance, evidence that they enhance strength or power is lacking. More important, they can be dangerous because large amounts of caffeine may cause serious heart and blood vessel problems such as heart rhythm disturbances and increases in heart rate and blood pressure. Caffeine also may harm children's still-developing cardiovascular and nervous systems. Caffeine use may be associated with palpitations, anxiety, sleep problems, digestive problems, elevated blood pressure, and dehydration.

In conclusion, if you want to follow a healthy, well balanced diet, make sure to pay attention not only to what you eat, but also to what you drink.

The Rocky Road to Adulthood

Growth and Pubertal Changes

A poster that hung in the endocrine section of a children's hospital read "Adolescence is hair-raising". This statement implies both the physical and the emotional changes of adolescence.

Puberty is a sequence of maturational events by which a child develops into an adult. Puberty occurs during adolescence and is the period during which complete growth, sexual maturity and fertility are achieved.

Puberty usually occurs in girls between the ages of 10 and 14 and in boys between the ages of 12 and 16. Nowadays, adolescent girls reach puberty at earlier ages than documented previously. In 1900, the average age of menarche (the first menstrual period) was 15; by the 1990s, this average had dropped to 12 and a half years of age. Many factors contribute to the timing of the onset of puberty, such as race, weight, body fat composition, nutritional status, heredity, and socioeconomic status. It appears that, in recent years, the increased incidence of childhood obesity may be related to the overall earlier onset of puberty.

While puberty involves a series of biological or physical transformations, the process can also affect the psychosocial and emotional development of the adolescent. As pre-teen girls and boys enter puberty they are confronted by changes, both in the way they look and in the way they feel.

The changes of puberty are the result of rising levels of hormones that lead to ovarian and testicular development. In girls, as the ovaries develop, estrogen and other hormones such as androgens, are produced leading to secondary sexual characteristics. The sequence of sexual changes in girls is breast development, uterine, vaginal, labial, and clitoral growth, pubic and axillary hair appearance, sweat gland enlargement, and menarche. Menarche, the onset of menstruation, usually occurs around two and a half years after the physical changes of puberty. Once a girl begins having menstrual periods, regular ovulation develops as well, marking the beginning of fertility. In boys, as the testicles develop, testosterone is produced, leading to secondary sexual characteristics. The sequence of sexual changes in boys is growth of the scrotum and testes, lengthening of the penis, appearance of pubic, axillary, and facial hair, and growth of the seminal vesicles and prostate. Boys go through spermarche (first ejaculation) at a mean age of thirteen. Mature spermatozoa appear between ages fourteen and sixteen leading to fertility, which is the ability to procreate.

During puberty, there is rapid increase in height, referred to as a growth spurt, which lasts for two to three years. The growth spurt typically occurs earlier in girls than in boys, with girls having the growth spurt on average two years prior to boys.

Common concerns in girls include problems with early or delayed onset of physical development and menstruation, irregular menses, breast size and height. Boys may be concerned about short stature, delayed appearance of facial hair, and genital size compared to their peers. Your physician can determine whether growth and development are progressing normally or whether studies may be necessary to exclude disease processes.

Puberty is accompanied by growth of bones, in length and width, and increases in bone density in both boys and girls. Since there is lag between bone growth and achievement of full bone density, adolescents may be at increased risk for fractures during this time.

Both boys and girls will start experiencing changes in weight and body composition. Adolescent girls develop a greater proportion of body fat than boys, while boys have a greater increase in muscle mass. As a result of that, by the end of puberty, boys have a muscle mass about one and a half times greater than that of comparably sized girls.

The physical signs of maturing can be exciting but also confusing and worrisome. Adolescence can also be hair-raising because of the changes in your feelings and moods. As your body changes, you need to get used to a new body image. The hormones may trigger changes in how you react to events and you may notice changes in your behavior. Both boys and girls can experience emotional changes that accompany the myriad physical changes of puberty. You may become irritated with parents, siblings, and friends, and feel happiness and sadness more intensely. You may experience mood swings and anxiety. Being aware of these changes is important for both you and the people close to you. If the emotional changes are unusually severe and start affecting your social life, or cause thoughts of harming yourself and/ or others, you need to talk to a health care professional.

Puberty is a normal condition and not an illness, but many medical conditions and illnesses may first appear during puberty. Some conditions potentially associated with puberty include the following: Acne: androgens, which are male hormones but are found in both men and women, cause excess oil to build up in the pores. When this oil clogs the pores it leads to the formation of comedones (whiteheads and blackheads) which may become infected with bacteria. This leads to the development of inflamed, red pimples that are seen in acne. The condition may vary from very mild and hardly noticeable to much more severe involving deeper tissues. This pustular form of acne may leave scarring of the skin of the face or back. Other factors that contribute to acne are stress, environment, genetics, and the use of certain cosmetics. Many treatments are available depending on the severity. Some medications reduce the build-up of excess oil, helping to unclog the pores. Other medications (antibiotics) fight the bacteria that cause infection. Some treatments are oral (by mouth) and some are topical (applied to the skin). Most people receive a combination of medications under the supervision of a physician. The most commonly used drugs include antibiotics, benzoyl peroxide, and retinoids. One of the most potent treatments is Accutane which is used only in more severe cases because of potentially harmful side effects and therefore requires close medical supervision. There is no evidence that greasy foods or chocolate cause acne. Non-comedogenic products should be used for skin care since make-up, sunscreens, and other facial products can aggravate acne. Squeezing pimples may cause permanent scarring. Acne can have a big impact on your emotional wellbeing. Our body image is influenced by the way others see us. Since acne is a disease of the face and skin, which everyone can see, it can have a big effect on body image for teen-agers. Acne has been associated with a wide range of psychological conditions, including depression, anxiety, and eating disorders.

Gynecomastia: gynecomastia is the term used to describe enlargement of the male breasts and affects up to one-half of normal adolescent boys. It's transient and can last for six to 18 months. Anemia: during puberty there is an increase in the ferritin (iron) and hemoglobin concentrations in males, but this increase is not seen in females. This, associated with the blood losses caused by menstrual bleeding, may place adolescent girls at risk for anemia.

Scoliosis: scoliosis, which is an abnormal curvature of the spine, can be worsened or may first develop during puberty.

Vision changes: nearsightedness (myopia) is common during puberty because of growth in the axial diameter of the eye.

Musculoskeletal injuries: we've already mention that adolescents are at risk for fractures, due to the fact that bone growth usually precedes full bone mineralization In addition to that, since the growth in the limbs usually occurs prior to growth in the trunk, some joints may have a limited range of motion, increasing the risk for sprains and strains.

Dysfunctional uterine bleeding: menstrual bleeding can be irregular heavy and prolonged, often due to anovulation (not ovulating). (http://www.medicinenet.com/puberty)

Sexual Concerns of Adolescents

Most sexual experimentation that involves risk-taking behavior occurs after menarche and spermarche. Early sexual experimentation may stem from the desire to be "grown-up". When one of the clear messages in the mass media is that intercourse is a rite of passage to adulthood and when many youth believe their peers to be sexually active, it is not a surprise that the "search for normalcy" results in sexual experimentation. Girls in particular are vulnerable to equating a sense of social belonging to providing sexual favors to adolescent boys and men regardless of whether the experience is healthy or pleasurable for them. Youth who feel disenfranchised from society, who believe that they have no meaningful future, may be much more cavalier about risking their health in multiple ways, including smoking, alcohol abuse, drug use and risky sexual behavior.

The range of sexual activity during adolescence is wide including exploration through talking with peers, reading forbidden magazines, fantasy, masturbation, and physical and sexual experimentation with the same and opposite gender peers. According to the US Centers for Disease Control and Prevention (CDC, www.cdc.gov), in the year 2007, 35% of US high school students were currently sexually active and 47.8% of US high school students reported having had sexual intercourse. Although there is a wide variability among youth influenced by class, race, and other factors, data show that the proportion of high school students who were sexually active has remained steady since 1997, approaching nearly 50% for all high school students with almost 70% of youth experiencing sexual intercourse by age 18. Approximately 7.1% of American youth report sexual intercourse prior to 13, with more male than female youth reporting early sexual debut; by age 16, approximately 30% of females and 34% of males have had sexual intercourse When youth, especially girls, have intercourse at an early age, particularly before the age of fifteen, there are detrimental consequences to both social development and physical health. There are several risk factors and protective factors related to sexual behaviors of adolescents. Risk factors for engaging in early sexual activity are male gender, history of abuse, substance abuse, poverty, belief that peers are sexually active and peer group pressure. Protective factors against early sexual activity are goals for the future, success in school, participation in extracurricular activities, involvement of concerned adults, and accurate information about sexuality.

Unprotected sexual intercourse is associated with a high risk of contracting sexually transmitted diseases such as HIV, Chlamydia, Gonorrhea, Trichomonas, Herpes and Syphilis, among others. The other risk of unprotected sexual intercourse is unplanned pregnancies, which carry many significant, negative consequences for young, adolescent women. They include dropping out of school, delayed social development, increased incidence of complications to both mother and baby, among others, as discussed in later chapters.

Sexual Orientation

The American Psychological Association (www. apa.org) defines sexual orientation as "our pattern of emotional, romantic and sexual attraction to another person". Sexual orientation exists along a continuum that ranges from exclusive heterosexuality to exclusive homosexuality and includes various forms of bisexuality. Bisexual persons experience sexual and emotional attraction to both their own and the opposite gender. Persons with a homosexual orientation are sometimes referred to as gay (both men arid women) or as lesbian (women only). Sexual orientation refers to feelings and self-concept. It may or may not be expressed in one's actual sexual behavior. In most people sexual orientation is shaped at an early age. There are numerous theories about the origin of a person's sexual orientation. Most scientists today agree that sexual orientation is most likely the result of a complex interaction of biological and environmental factors. There is considerable evidence to suggest that biology, including genetic or inborn hormonal factors, play a significant role in a person's sexuality. It is important to recognize that there are probably many reasons for a person's sexual orientation and the reason may be different for different people. Sexual orientation emerges for most people in early adolescence without any prior sexual experience. Although we can choose whether or not to act on our feelings, psychologists do not consider sexual orientation to be a conscious choice that can be changed voluntarily. Psychologists, psychiatrists, and other mental health professionals agree that homosexuality is not an illness, a mental disorder, or an emotional problem. Decades of scientific research has shown that homosexuality is not associated with mental disorders or emotional or social problems. Homosexuality was once considered to be a mental illness because mental health professionals and society had biased information. In the past the studies of gay, lesbian, and bisexual people involved only those in psychotherapy, thus biasing the resulting conclusions. As early as 1973 the American Psychiatric Association (www.psychiatry.org) confirmed the importance of new, better designed research, and removed homosexuality from the official list of mental and emotional disorders. The American Psychiatric Association and the American Psychological Association have urged all mental health professionals' to help dispel the stigma of mental illness that some still associate with homosexual orientation. Studies comparing children raised by homosexual and heterosexual parents find no developmental differences between the two groups of children in four critical areas: intelligence, psychological adjustment, social adjustment, and popularity with friends. It is also very important to realize that a parent's sexual orientation does not dictate that of the child. Often gay, lesbian, and bisexual people feel afraid, different, and alone when they first realize that their sexual orientation differs from the community norm. This is particularly true when people become aware of their gay, lesbian, or bisexual orientation as children or adolescents. Depending on their family and where they live, they may have to struggle against prejudice and misinformation about homosexuality. Children and adolescents may be particularly vulnerable to the deleterious effects of bias and stereotypes. They may also fear being rejected by family, friends, coworkers, and religious institutions. Some gay people have to worry about losing their jobs or being harassed and bullied at school if their sexual orientation were to become known. Unfortunately, despite recent progress, gay, lesbian, and bisexual people are at higher risk for hate crime, from name–calling to physical assault and violence than are heterosexual.

Some states include violence against an individual on the basis of his/her sexual orientation as a hate crime and there are laws against discrimination on the basis of sexual orientation.

Research has found that people who know homosexual individuals as friends or colleagues have the most positive attitude toward them. For this reason psychologists believe that a negative attitude is not grounded in actual experience but is based on stereotype and prejudice.

Education about homosexuality is likely to diminish anti-gay prejudice. Accurate information is especially important to young people who are first discovering and seeking to understand their sexuality. Fear that access to such information will make more people gay has no validity. Information about homosexuality does not determine one's sexual orientation. On the contrary, lack of education about the nature of sexuality, conservative religious doctrines, and many people's innate or learned fear of what is foreign to their experience promotes continued prejudice and hostility.

An Extreme Gamble: Drug Use

Illegal drug use crosses all boundaries of sex, age, race, and socioeconomic status (National Institute on Drug Abuse, www.drugabuse.gov; CDC, www.cdc.gov; National Survey on Drugs and Health, https://nsduhweb. rti.org; Substance Abuse and Mental Health Services Administration, www.samhsa.gov). Here are some frightening facts: drug users have a higher incidence of sexually transmitted diseases and poor nutrition which makes them at higher risk for other diseases. Sharing needles increases the risk of acquiring infections such as HIV which causes AIDS, and hepatitis B and C. In addition, illegal drugs taken during pregnancy may lead to premature birth or death of the fetus. If the baby survives, he/she may already be addicted to the drug and may be born with physical and mental deficits. IV (intravenous) drug use is a major public health problem. According to the World Drug Report published by the United Nations Office on Drugs and Crime (UNODC, www. unodc.org) for the year 2015, there were an estimated 12 million injection drug users worldwide. People who inject drugs are considered the most marginalized among those who use drugs. Injection of illegal drugs causes several health hazards and complications. Chronic users will have needle marks or scars at the site of injections. Long term users are usually forced to seek new injection sites as old sites become unusable because of scarring. Skin and soft tissue infections are very common. The damaged skin becomes colonized with organisms that cause superficial or deep infections. The types of infection include cellulitis, abscesses, multiple chronic ulcerations, phlebitis, and necrotizing fasciitis. Local lymphadenopathy (swollen glands) is common with all these conditions.

Symptoms of cellulitis, a skin infection commonly caused by Staphylococcus (staph) Aureus, include red streaking of the skin, pain, swelling, tenderness, swollen lymph nodes, leakage of yellow fluid from blisters and fever. Treatments for cellulitis include oral antibiotics and elevation of the affected areas. Severe cellulitis may require a hospital admission for intravenous antibiotics.

If staph spreads to the lungs, it can produce symptoms of pneumonia, such as cough with yellow or green sputum, chest pain when breathing or coughing, elevated fever and chills. This condition can be life threatening and requires hospitalization for intravenous antibiotics and life support measures.

Abscesses are pus filled masses surrounded by red, inflamed skin. Abscesses may drain on their own, but most of the times they need to be opened and drained surgically, as they won't respond to antibiotic treatment, if left intact. If the infection spreads, it might cause fever/chills, malaise, nausea/vomiting and lead to hospitalization for further treatment.

Necrotizing fasciitis is a serious bacterial disease and can develop quickly. The name comes from the Latin "necro," meaning "death," as this disease causes death of the skin and the tissues beneath the skin. When the bacteria spread, gangrene develops and the skin blackens.

If the infection is not treated promptly, it may spread to the internal organs and lead to death. Treatments may include surgery to remove the dead tissues or perform amputation, intravenous antibiotics, hyperbaric oxygen therapy and hospitalization in an intensive care unit.

Botulism is caused by a bacterial toxin, with resulting flaccid paralysis of muscles, blurry vision, dry mouth, difficulty swallowing, slurred speech and drooping eyelids, among other symptoms. Severe botulism can cause respiratory failure and death. Botulism is treated using antitoxins to counteract the neurotoxins in the blood.

Tetanus may develop when the spores of the Clostridium Tetani bacteria enter the bloodstream through an open wound from an intravenous injection site. Symptoms include generalized muscle spasms resulting in painful arching of the back and lockjaw. Other symptoms include difficulty breathing and swallowing, drooling, fever and irritability. Tetanus immunoglobulin, antibiotics, muscle relaxers, sedatives and bed rest are the available treatments for tetanus.

Septic thrombophlebitis is a bacterial infection of a blood vessel, characterized by a tender, swollen vein, overlaid by red, inflamed skin. If the infection spreads to the blood stream, sepsis may develop, with resulting drop in blood pressure, difficulty breathing, rapid heart rate, altered mental status and even coma. Treatments for septic thrombophlebitis include intravenous antibiotics, non-steroidal anti-inflammatory drugs, anticoagulants and, if necessary, surgery to remove the infected vein.

Bacterial endocarditis (BE), which may lead to valve destruction and heart failure, is an infection of the heart valve caused by bacteria spreading through the bloodstream and colonizing the heart valves. BE symptoms include fever, chills, night sweats, chest pain, back pain, abdominal pain, muscle aches, weakness, malaise, weight loss and shortness of breath. Septic emboli, small pieces of infected material, may detach from the valve and travel through the blood stream, setting up infections in other organs, especially in the lungs (pneumonia). Treatment for this disease includes intravenous antibiotics and, when required, heart surgery to repair or replace affected heart valves.

Ophthalmic complications (endophtalmitis) are also seen in IV drug users such as bacterial or mycotic infection of the eyes. Osteomyelitis, infection of the bone, and septic arthritis, infection of a joint, occur mainly by spread of a bacteria through the blood stream.

Other complications related to intravenous drug use include HIV transmission and Hepatitis.

The risk for getting or transmitting HIV is very high if an HIV-negative person uses injection equipment that someone with HIV has used. This high risk is because the drug materials may have blood in them, and blood can carry HIV.

In 2015, 10% of the HIV in the United States were attributed to IDU and another 3% to male-to-male sexual contact and IDU.

Of the HIV diagnoses attributed to IDU, 59% were among men, 41% were among women, 38% were among blacks/African Americans, 40% were among whites, and 19% were among Hispanics/Latinos. Risk estimates show that the average chance that an HIV-negative person will get HIV from sharing needles with an HIV-positive person is about 1 in 160.

Injecting drugs can reduce inhibition and increase risky sexual behavior, such as having unprotected sex, or having sex with multiple partners, or trading sex for money or drugs, which, of course, can increase the risk of contracting HIV.

Social and economic factors, such as being homeless, not having health insurance, being incarcerated, mistrust of the health care system and stigma associated with drug use, may limit access to HIV prevention and treatment services among intravenous drug users, further contributing to the spread of HIV.

In addition to being at risk for HIV, IV drug users can get other serious health problems, like Hepatitis B virus (HBV) and Hepatitis C virus (HCV), which may be easily transmitted, not only through sharing needles, but also trough paraphernalia used in the preparation of the drugs. The sexual route is another very common source of infection. Both Hepatitis B and C may cause liver failure, cirrhosis, liver cancer and death. In fact, HBV and HCV infections are the major risk factors for liver cancer worldwide, an estimated 22,000 people are expected to die from this disease in 2013 in the United States alone, a number that has been steadily increasing over the past several years. During the next 40–50 years, 1 million people with untreated chronic HCV infection will likely die from complications related to their HCV. Viral hepatitis may be tricky to diagnose and treat because the vast majority of people who have it show no symptoms. However, some telltale signs and symptoms of this disease include extreme fatigue, itchy skin, sore muscles, dark urine and stomach pain that may be accompanied by bleeding and jaundice (yellowing of the skin or eyes).

The association of drug use and hepatitis A has been recognized only recently. Two possible explanations for the association between hepatitis A and drug use have been proposed: 1) HAV (hepatitis A virus) may be transmitted by injection or ingestion of contaminated drugs or 2) transmission may result from direct person-to-person contact. Drugs could become contaminated with fecal material containing HAV at the cultivation site (e.g., through use of human feces as fertilizer) or during transport, preparation, or distribution (e.g., through smuggling in condoms concealed in the rectum).

Person-to-person transmission of HAV between drug abusers could result from sharing needles, from sexual contact, or from generally poor sanitary and personal hygiene conditions, which have often been observed among drug abusers.

An additional risk of illegal drugs lies in the uncertainty regarding the actual ingredients in the product. Other toxic materials may have been mixed with the specific drug causing unexpected, deadly consequences. Since one cannot know the exact amount of pure drug being taken, it is impossible to predict the intensity of the reaction and fatal outcomes occur.

Opiods

The terms opiates and narcotics are sometimes encountered as synonyms for opioids. The term narcotics it is also loosely applied to any illegal or controlled psychoactive drug. In some jurisdictions all controlled drugs are legally classified as narcotics.

Opioids are a class of drugs that include the illegal drug heroin, synthetic opioids such as fentanyl, and pain relievers available legally by prescription, such as oxycodone (OxyContin), hydrocodone (Vicodin), codeine, morphine, and many others. These drugs are chemically related and interact with opioid receptors on nerve cells in the body and brain. Opioid pain relievers are generally safe when taken for a short time and as prescribed by a doctor, but because they produce euphoria in addition to pain relief, they can be misused (taken in a different way or in a larger quantity than prescribed, or taken without a doctor's prescription). Regular use, even as prescribed by a doctor, can lead to dependence and, when misused, opioid pain relievers can lead to overdose incidents and deaths.

The abuse of and addiction to opioids such as heroin, morphine, and prescription pain relievers is a serious global problem that affects the health, social, and economic welfare of all societies. It is estimated that between 26.4 million and 36 million people abuse opioids worldwide, with an estimated 2.1 million people in the United States suffering from substance use disorders related to prescription opioid pain relievers in 2012 and an estimated 467,000 addicted to heroin. The consequences of this abuse have been devastating and are on the rise. For example, the number of unintentional overdose deaths from prescription pain relievers has soared in the United States, more than quadrupling since 1999. There is also growing evidence to suggest a relationship between increased non-medical use of opioid analgesics and heroin abuse in the United States.

Opioids dull the senses, relieve pain, and produce sleep. The most familiar of the illegal narcotics is heroin. Addiction to heroin develops quickly, and chronic use causes serious health problems. Heroin is usually injected intravenously, but can also be injected intramuscularly or subcutaneously (skin popping) or sniffed (snorting). The effect after intravenous injection consists of a brief, intense period of euphoria followed by several hours of a "pleasant, dreamy state". The skin may itch due to histamine release which leads to characteristic scratching. Immediate side effects include increase talkativeness, red eyes, increased motor activity, vomiting, constricted pupils, and respiratory depression. The respiratory depression may be severe and may lead to death.

Complications related to long term heroin use include kidney damage and brain damage such as a severe form of Parkinsonism. Tolerance is a condition in which the person starts craving higher dosages of heroin to obtain the same effect. The lack of the drug causes withdrawal symptoms, such as anxiety, nausea, diarrhea, sweating, dilated pupils, "goose flesh", otherwise called piloerection. The craving is so intense, it may drive the person to criminal activity to continue the habit. In an attempt to deal with the addiction to this illegal drug, methadone clinics were developed. Methadone, a synthetic substitute for heroin, is given to individuals addicted to heroin to help them function in society without heroine. Patients maintained on methadone become both physically and psychologically dependent on this drug as well. Many experience considerable difficulty making the transition from methadone to abstinence. Some patients who make appropriate changes in life style and develop good social and emotional support systems are able to detoxify from methadone successfully (https://www.drugabuse.gov).

Stimulants

Cocaine is one of the most commonly abused stimulant drugs. Cocaine is used in several forms. The route for cocaine intake depends upon the form used. The natural water soluble powder is either sniffed (snorted) and absorbed through the nasal mucosa, or is injected intravenously. Forms of cocaine that can be smoked are produced by extracting or "freeing" the cocaine alkaloid from the hydrochloride salt. The resulting product is referred to as "free base". When baking soda and water are used as reagents the resulting product is "crack", so named because of the cracking sound that is produced when the drug is smoked. Cocaine quickly produces a short but intense feeling of well-being, increasing self-confidence, and sexual stimulation. Other effects include increased heart rate, dilated pupils, and increased body temperature. The capacity to produce euphoria gives cocaine a high abuse potential. The physical effects of cocaine put a strain on the body that can lead to hypertension, arrhythmia, stroke, seizure, convulsions, and heart attacks even in young people without other risk factors for heart disease. High doses of cocaine may also cause respiratory depression and death. Chronic use of cocaine, amphetamines, or other long acting stimulants causes initial hyperactivity and irritability followed by lethargy and depression. People can also develop sleep disturbances, weight loss, emotional lability and organic delusional disorders that resemble paranoid schizophrenia.

Methamphetamine is a man-made stimulant drug, a more potent form of the drug amphetamine.

There are different forms of methamphetamine, generally distinguished by their appearance and perceived purity.

The three main forms are: crystalline (ice or crystal), powder (speed) and base.

Methamphetamine is a stimulant drug usually used as a white, bitter-tasting powder or a pill. Crystal methamphetamine is a form of the drug that looks like glass fragments or shiny, bluish-white rocks. It is chemically similar to amphetamine, a drug used to treat attention-deficit hyperactivity disorder (ADHD) and narcolepsy, a sleep disorder.

Other common names for methamphetamine include chalk, crank, crystal, ice, meth, and speed.

People can take methamphetamine by inhaling/ smoking, swallowing (pill), snorting, injecting the powder that has been dissolved in water/alcohol.

Because the high from the drug both starts and fades quickly, people often take repeated doses in a "binge and crash" pattern. In some cases, people take methamphetamine in a form of binging known as a "run", giving up food and sleep while continuing to take the drug every few hours for up to several days.

Methamphetamine increases the amount of the natural chemical dopamine in the brain. Dopamine is involved in body movement, motivation, pleasure, and reward (pleasure from natural behaviors such as eating). The drug's ability to release high levels of dopamine rapidly in reward areas of the brain produces the "rush" (euphoria) or "flash" that many people experience.

Short-Term, taking even small amounts of methamphetamine can result in many of the same health effects as those of other stimulants, such as cocaine or amphetamines. These include:

increased wakefulness and physical activity, decreased appetite, faster breathing, rapid and/or irregular heartbeat, increased blood pressure and body temperature.

The use of these drugs may cause heart attacks, strokes and death. Long-term use can lead to brain and liver damage, kidney and lung problems, psychological disorders and behavioral changes resembling paranoid schizophrenia (www.drugabuse.gov).

Amphetamine is a potent stimulant of the central nervous system (CNS), which causes emotional and cognitive changes. At therapeutic doses, it's used in the treatment of a variety of medical conditions, including attention deficit hyperactivity disorder (ADHD), narcolepsy and obesity, due to its ability to increase wakefulness and cognitive control, decrease reaction time, improve fatigue resistance and muscle strength. Larger doses of amphetamine though may impair cognitive function, induce rapid muscle breakdown, cause psychosis, delusions and paranoia, which rarely occurs at therapeutic doses even during long-term use. (https://chem.libretexts.org).

Hallucinogens

Hallucinogenic drugs include cannabis (marijuana/ hashish), LSD (lysergic acid diethylamide), and PCP (phencyclidine) commonly called angel dust. These drugs affect the central nervous system and distort one's view of reality leading to self-endangerment. PCP causes a state of sensory deprivation with relative wakefulness that creates a peculiar sense of detachment, disembodiment, and feeling of weightlessness. These sensations may be intensely pleasurable for some, whereas for others, they may induce intense anxiety and panic. Street names for PCP vary considerably from region to region, but it is most commonly known as angel dust, flakes, crystal, or sheets. PCP may cause a severe reaction leading to delirium and violence. High doses of PCP can result in coma, respiratory depression, seizure, and death. Chronic use of PCP may produce changes in personal habits (hygiene or dress), memory loss, speech and sleep disturbances, mood changes, and paranoid thinking. Little is known about long-term physical effects.

LSD is sold in the form of powder, tablets, or capsules and is usually ingested by mouth. LSD causes slight increase in blood pressure and heart rate, increased salivation, lacrimation, and dilated pupils. LSD may produce body image distortion, labile mood, altered time perception, and vivid_flashbacks.

Marijuana is derived from dried leaves of the cannabis plant. Hashish is a concentrated resin of cannabis containing five to ten times the amount of the principal psychoactive ingredient (tetrahydrocannabinol, THC) as does marijuana. The effects of marijuana include a sense of euphoria with increased tendency to laughter and silliness, tachycardia, red eyes, and, later, relaxation. At higher doses, all these effects are enhanced. The drug may distort the perception of sound, color, and other sensations. It impairs short term memory, logical thinking, and the ability to perform complex tasks. Thus, the ability to drive may be seriously impaired. The most frequent adverse response to marijuana is acute anxiety and paranoid ideation. As far as chronic adverse effects, there is evidence that marijuana use may result in impaired memory, apathy, and a loss of energy and drive. There is evidence that marijuana reduces testosterone levels in men. It has also been reported that marijuana smoke contains more carcinogens that does tobacco smoke. Although there is a reason for concern, there are no data yet which demonstrate an association of cancer with marijuana. Cannabis has effects that are potentially useful for therapeutic purposes, such as the ability to decrease intra-ocular pressure and anti-emetic properties. The term medical marijuana refers to using the whole, unprocessed marijuana plant or its basic extracts to treat symptoms of illness and other conditions. The U.S. Food and Drug Administration (FDA) has not recognized or approved the marijuana plant as medicine.

However, scientific study of the chemicals in marijuana, called cannabinoids, has led to two FDA-approved medications that contain cannabinoid chemicals in pill form. Continued research may lead to more medications.

Because the marijuana plant contains chemicals that may help treat a range of illnesses and symptoms, many people argue that it should be legal for medical purposes. In fact, a growing number of states have legalized marijuana for medical use. Significant changes have taken place in the policy landscape surrounding cannabis legalization, production, and use. During the past 20 years, 25 states and the District of Columbia have legalized cannabis and/or cannabidiol (a component of cannabis) for medical conditions or retail sales at the state level and 4 states have legalized both the medical and recreational use of cannabis. The FDA requires carefully conducted studies (clinical trials) in hundreds to thousands of human subjects to determine the benefits and risks of a possible medication. So far, researchers haven't conducted enough large-scale clinical trials that show that the benefits of the marijuana plant (as opposed to its cannabinoid ingredients) outweigh its risks in patients it's meant to treat (http://strengthheal. us/drugfacts-is-marijuana-medicine).

Synthetic marijuana/Kush:

Synthetic marijuana and synthetic cannabinoids are a family of synthetic, man-made chemicals capable of interacting with the same cell receptors in the brain as THC, the active ingredient in natural cannabis. These chemicals are sprayed onto diced-up dry leaves/plant material that is sold in baggies and smoked as traditional marijuana. When you buy synthetic marijuana, you don't really know which chemical you're inhaling.

Spice and K2 refer to the same kind of products. Other names that have been used include Bliss, Cowboy Kush, and Scooby Snax. Goofy images of dragons, smiley faces, and cartoon animals are common on the packaging, which makes them even more appealing to young people. (http://www.slate.com/articles/)

Inhalants/Solvent Abuse

The inhalation of solvents is a form of substance abuse that is common among children and adolescents. Solvents are easily obtained and inexpensive. Examples of these substances include gasoline, glue, spray paint, lighter fluid, nail polish remover, shoe polish, and cleaning fluids. Chemicals such as toluene are the active components that cause the "high". Inhalation is achieved by saturating a rag with the substance and holding it directly over the face or by placing it in a bag that is then placed over the nose and the mouth. The effects of solvents are immediate and short acting, usually disappearing in just a few hours. They may be similar to alcohol intoxication. Common acute adverse effects are headache, nausea, occasional delirium, and body image distortions. Users can also experience nosebleeds and lose their sense of hearing or smell. Chronic use can lead to muscle wasting and reduced muscle tone, and the poisonous chemicals gradually damage the lungs and the immune system. An inhalant user risks Sudden Sniffing Death Syndrome. Death can occur the first time or the hundredth time an inhalant is used and is usually from cardiac arrhythmia. Inhalant use can cause damage to the heart, kidneys, brain, liver, bone marrow and other organs. Cerebellar damage and peripheral neuropathy may also occur with long-term use. Chronic solvent abuse requires intensive counseling and rehabilitative intervention. (http://www.drugfreeworld.org/drugfacts/inhalants/how-do-inhalants-affect-your-body.html)

Date Rape Drugs

A date rape drug, also referred to as a predator drug, is any drug that is an incapacitating agent which, when administered to another person, incapacitates the person and renders them vulnerable to a drug facilitated sexual assault (DFSA), including rape. The most common types of DFSA are those in which a victim consumes a recreational drug such as alcohol administered surreptitiously. The most common form of DFSA is alcohol-related, with the victim in most cases consuming the alcohol voluntarily. Other date rape drugs include ecstasy, gamma-hydroxybutyrate (GHB), rohypnol and ketamine. (https://en.wikipedia.org/wiki/Date_rape_drug)

Ecstasy

Street names: X, Lover's speed, Clarity, Adams and others

Ecstasy is an amphetamine-like substance with the chemical name of methylenedioxymethamphetamine (MDMA) that was first widely used during the 1970's to assist patients in opening up to psychiatrists during therapy. By the end of the decade, the drug reached the dance floor in the discos throughout the country. In 1985, ecstasy was made illegal in this country and subject to criminal penalties similar to those for cocaine and heroine. Ecstasy usually comes in a pill form. Ecstasy causes a feeling of happiness and disinhibition. It became associated with certain behaviors like sex and dancing. It is a popular drug at raves, all night teen dance parties, where it is known as the 'hug' drug because it causes the teens to lose restraint in touching one another. It is a popular drug among teenagers during 'spring break' gatherings. Users consider ecstasy harmless but the drug is thought to be habit-forming. Whether or not the drug is addictive, ecstasy does affect the ability to concentrate and make competent decisions. Users may experience deep depression after using the drug. The depression following the initial high may actually last longer than the users think. Over time an increasing amount of ecstasy may be needed to reach a high.

GHB

Gamma-hydroxybutyrate (GHB) is an illegal substance that has recently gained popularity among body-builders and party-goers. GHB is most commonly found in a clear liquid form that tastes slightly salty. There are at least thirty street names to refer to GHB: "G" (most common), Gamma-OH, Liquid E, Fantasy, Georgia Home Boy, Grievous Bodily Harm, Liquid X, Liquid Ecstasy (is not ecstasy), Scoop, Water, Everclear, Great Hormones at Bedtime, GBH, Soap, Easy Lay, Salty Water, G-Riffick, Cherry Meth, and Organic Quaalude, Jib.

Persons who attend nightclubs and parties (such as all-night "raves) use it as a euphoriant and aphrodisiac. Effects vary considerably among individuals without any predictability.

Effects include intoxication, increased energy, happiness, talking, desire to socialize, feeling affectionate and playful, mild disinhibition, sensuality, enhanced sexual experience, muscle relaxation, loss of coordination due to loss of muscle tone, possible nausea, difficulty concentrating, loss of gag reflex. Many people have bad reactions. These can include nausea, headaches, drowsiness, dizziness, amnesia, vomiting, hallucinations, seizures, aggression, loss of muscle control, respiratory problems, loss of consciousness, being conscious but unable to move, and death, especially when combined with alcohol or other drugs. (http://www.trendydrugs.org/what_is_ghb.htm)

Rohypnol

Street names: Roofies, Roach, Forget-Me pill and others

Rohypnol (flunitrazepam) belongs to a class of drugs known as benzodiazepines. It's not approved for use in the United States. It is commonly found as white tablets that dissolve easily in carbonated beverages. The tablets can also be grounded up for snorting. Rohypnol is sometimes taken to enhance a heroin high, or to mellow or ease the experience of coming down from a cocaine or crack high. Rohypnol causes drowsiness, visual disturbances, difficulty with motor movements and speech, confusion and amnesia, which is the inability to remember events that happened while under the influence of the drug. When used in combination with alcohol, the risk of coma and death are high due to respiratory depression.

Ketamine

Street names: Special K, "vitamin K", super K and others

Ketamine is a drug used by veterinarians (animal doctors) as a tranquilizer. It is chemically similar to PCP. Ketamine is available in a liquid form and in a powder form. The powder is usually snorted or smoked with marijuana or tobacco. It can be injected, consumed in drinks, snorted, or added to joints or cigarettes. Ketamine was placed on the list of controlled substances in the US in 1999. Short- and long-term effects include increased heart rate and blood pressure, nausea, vomiting, numbness, depression, amnesia, hallucinations and potentially fatal respiratory problems. Ketamine users can also develop cravings for the drug. At high doses, users experience an effect referred to as "K-Hole," an "out of body" or "near-death" experience.

Due to the detached, dreamlike state it creates, where the user finds it difficult to move, ketamine has been used as a "date-rape" drug. (http://www.drugfreeworld. org/drugfacts/prescription/ketamine.html)

Dextromethorphan (DXM)

DXM is a drug related to morphine that doctors might prescribe to suppress the cough reflex in their patients. It has become another of the so-called 'recreational' drugs. Abusers experience loss of motor control and loss of touch with reality. These effects are similar to those of alcohol, marijuana, and PCP. DXM is an ingredient in many over-the-counter cough and cold remedies. It is safe when taken at the recommended dosage. Some teenagers, however, looking for a quick 'high' often take double doses at a time. They may also mix it with alcohol and other drugs which may be deadly. Unpleasant side effects include upset stomach, vomiting, itching, diarrhea, fast heart rate, and red blotchy skin.

Alcohol Use

Alcohol use is risky. While adults may enjoy alcoholic beverages in small amounts in social situations, alcohol in larger amounts will decrease inhibitions and depress the central nervous system. Depending on the individual's blood alcohol level, there is danger of sedation, lack of coordination, delirium and ultimately loss of consciousness and death. Alcohol abuse may cause immediate health problems and complications, such as bleeding and inflammation in the stomach (gastritis), inflammation of the pancreas (pancreatitis), and inflammation of the liver (hepatitis).

The long-term health hazards of alcohol include damage to the liver (cirrhosis), brain, nerves and heart. With the loss of inhibition and control there is the increased likelihood of behavior leading to injury to self and others. Examples include car crashes, unplanned and risky sexual activity, and date rape (National Institute on Alcohol Abuse and Alcoholism, www.niaaa.nih.gov).

Harmful and underage college drinking are significant public health problems, and they exact an enormous toll on the intellectual and social lives of students on campuses across the United States.

Drinking at college has become a ritual that students often see as an integral part of their higher education experience. Many students come to college with established drinking habits, and the college environment can exacerbate the problem. According to a national survey, almost 60 percent of college students ages 18–22 drank alcohol in the past month, 1 and almost 2 out of 3 of them engaged in binge drinking during that same timeframe. About 20 percent of college students meet the criteria for an alcohol use disorder (AUD).

According to the "Dietary Guidelines for Americans 2015-2020," U.S. Department of Health and Human Services (www.hhs.gov) and U.S. Department of Agriculture (www.usda.gov), moderate drinking is up to 1 drink per day for women and up to 2 drinks per day for men.

Binge Drinking is defined by The National Institute on Alcohol Abuse and Alcoholism (NIAAA) as a pattern of drinking that brings blood alcohol concentration (BAC) levels to 0.08 g/dL. This typically occurs after 4 drinks for women and 5 drinks for men, in about 2 hours.

The Substance Abuse and Mental Health Services Administration (SAMHSA www.samhsa.gov), which conducts the annual National Survey on Drug Use and Health (NSDUH https://nsduhweb.rti.org), defines binge drinking as 5 or more alcoholic drinks for males or 4 or more alcoholic drinks for females on the same occasion (i.e., at the same time or within a couple of hours of each other) on at least 1 day in the past month.

Heavy Alcohol Use is defined by SAMHSA as binge drinking on 5 or more days in the past month.

Drinking affects college students, their families, and college communities at large. Researchers estimate that each year:

- about 1,825 college students between the ages of 18 and 24 die from alcohol-related unintentional injuries, including motor-vehicle crashes.
- about 696,000 students between the ages of 18 and 24 are assaulted by another student who has been drinking.
- about 97,000 students between the ages of 18 and 24 report experiencing alcohol-related sexual assault or date rape.
- about 1 in 4 college students reported academic consequences from drinking, including missing class, falling behind in class, doing poorly on exams or papers, and receiving lower grades overall.5 In a national survey of college students, binge drinkers who consumed alcohol at least 3 times per week were roughly 6 times more likely than those who drank but never binged to perform poorly on a test or project as a result of drinking (40 percent vs. 7 percent) and 5 times more likely to have missed a class (64 percent vs. 12 percent).

Other consequences include suicide attempts, health problems, injuries, unsafe sex, and driving under the influence of alcohol, as well as vandalism, property damage, and involvement with the police.

From 1976 to 1983, several states voluntarily raised their purchase ages to 19 (or, less commonly, 20 or 21), in part to combat drunk driving fatalities. In 1984, Congress passed the National Minimum Drinking Age Act, which required states to raise their ages for purchase and public possession to 21 by October 1986 or lose 10% of their federal highway funds. By mid-1988, all 50 states and the District of Columbia had raised their purchase ages to 21 (but not Puerto Rico, Guam, or the Virgin Islands). The current drinking age of 21 remains a point of contention among many Americans, because of it being higher than the age of majority (18 in most states) and higher than the drinking ages of most other countries. (https://en.wikipedia.org/wiki/U.S._history_of_alcohol_minimum_purchase_age_by_state)

For the most part, DUI (Driving Under the Influence) or DWI (Driving While Intoxicated) are synonymous terms that represent the criminal offense of operating (or in some jurisdictions merely being in physical control of) a motor vehicle while being under the influence of alcohol or drugs or a combination of both. Laboratory tests and roadside breathalyzers have been developed for the purpose of detecting the level of a controlled substance in an individual's body.

Every state in the U.S. designates a blood or breath alcohol level as the threshold point for an independent criminal offense. On May 14, 2013, the National Transportation Safety Board recommended that all 50 states lower the benchmark for determining when a driver is legally drunk from 0.08 % or greater blood-alcohol content (units of milligrams per deciliter, representing 8 g of alcohol in 10 liters of blood) to 0.05. The idea is part of an initiative to eliminate drunk driving, which accounts for about a third of all road deaths.

Certain people should avoid alcohol completely, including those who plan to drive a vehicle or operate machinery, take medications that interact with alcohol, have a medical condition that alcohol can aggravate, are pregnant or trying to become pregnant

Tobacco

There is now extensive evidence of the harmful consequences of tobacco use, whether in the form of cigarette smoking or chewing tobacco. The danger results from nicotine and other compounds present in tobacco smoke. Of the more than 7,000 chemicals in tobacco smoke, at least 250 are known to be harmful, including hydrogen cyanide, carbon monoxide, and ammonia. Among the 250 known harmful chemicals in tobacco smoke, at least 69 can cause cancer. Nicotine dependence is considered a substance use disorder by the American Psychiatric Association with similar features to those of alcoholism and drug abuse. Smoking begins in the pre-teen or teenage years. Young people may start smoking because of peer pressure and the mistaken idea that smoking makes them appear independent, mature and self-confident. Teenagers may also mimic the habits of their parents.

Nicotine dependence, also referred to as tobacco dependence, is an addiction to tobacco products caused by the drug nicotine. Nicotine is the chemical agent responsible for the development of the addiction to tobacco use.

Nicotine produces physical and mood-altering effects in your brain that are temporarily pleasing. These effects make you want to use tobacco and lead to dependence. Dependence means you can't easily quit, as stopping tobacco use causes withdrawal symptoms, such as physical malaise, irritability and anxiety. The nicotine in tobacco is responsible for nicotine dependence, but the toxic effects of tobacco result from other substances in tobacco. Smoking can significantly shorten life expectancy, as smokers have much higher rates of heart disease, hypertension, stroke and cancer than nonsmokers do. (http://www.recoveryhealth.org/sarah.php?cid=6&pid=100). Smoking is also associated with an increased risk of emphysema, osteoporosis, and many types of cancer including cancer of the lungs, mouth, throat, pancreas, esophagus, bladder, prostate, and cervix. In addition to that, when used during pregnancy smoking is also associated with increased risk of early delivery and stillbirth. Smokeless tobacco is not risk free, Smokeless tobacco include chewing or spit tobacco, snuff or dipping tobacco and dissolvable tobacco in the form of lozenges, orbs, pellets and strips. People who dip or chew tobacco get about the same amount of nicotine as regular smokers. They also get at least 30 chemicals that are known to cause cancer. The most harmful cancer-causing substances in smokeless tobacco are tobacco-specific nitrosamines (TSNAs). TSNA levels vary by product, but the higher the level the greater the cancer risk.

Tobacco stains teeth and causes bad breath. It can also irritate or destroy gum tissue. Many regular smokeless tobacco users have receding gums, gum disease, cavities and tooth decay (from the high sugar content in the tobacco), scratching and wearing down (abrasion) of teeth, and bone loss around the teeth. The surface of the tooth root may be exposed where gums have shrunken. All this can cause teeth to loosen and fall out.

Teenagers who smoke are much more likely to suffer from depression and anxiety disorders. Smoking low-yield cigarettes does not reduce the health risks. If you have begun smoking, it is important for you to seek medical assistance to aid in quitting this unsafe habit.

Supplements: How Much is too Much?

In the past decade, there has been an increasing public enthusiasm regarding herbal and non-herbal supplements. Some of the most commonly used herbal supplements include Soy, Garlic, Gingko, Echinacea, Milk thistle, Black cohosh and St. John's Wort. Non-herbal supplements include vitamins, minerals, amino acids and hormones. Herbal supplements are beyond the scope of this chapter. We'll focus on non-herbal supplements, particularly on those believed to enhance athletic performance.

Sports Supplements

Sports supplements are becoming increasingly popular among adolescents, sports enthusiasts, body builders, and weight lifters. Many people consider herbs and nutritional supplements to be safe "because they are natural". People may not consider the possible adverse effects of such substances when taken alone or in combination with other medications. Besides protein supplements, there are several sports supplements used to enhance performance. Many adolescents use a number of sports supplements such as creatine, DHEA (dehydroepiandrosterone), and androstenedione.

Androstenedione was marketed as a natural alternative to anabolic steroids and was used to increase the serum testosterone levels and promote muscle growth.

On April 11, 2004, the United States Food and Drug Administration banned the sale of Δ4-dione (androstenedione), citing that the drug poses significant health risks commonly associated with steroids. The side effects for men include breast development, behavioral changes, heart disease, and more. Additionally, a study done on an individual links androstenedione intake with priapism in men. Side effects for women are similar to the side effects from anabolic steroids in that their voices will deepen and they may grow facial hair since both occur from an increase level of testosterone. Another side effect of Δ4-dione is male-pattern baldness. The main psychological side effect of Δ4-dione is depression. Mood swings are also common of any user. A 2007 study showed that androstenedione has detrimental effects on endothelial cells in vitro, as a 400 μM concentration was able to kill half of the cells.

Δ4-Dione is currently banned by the U.S. military.

In addition, supraphysiologic levels of testosterone in adolescents can cause premature maturation of the long bones with decreased height in adulthood. Increased levels of serum testosterone have also been associated with an increased risk of cardiovascular disease which may result from changes in the cholesterol level.

The manufacturers of creatine claim that their product improves muscle strength, endurance, and lean body weight. Creatine is formed by the liver and the kidneys and is also found in meat and fish. A 2003 study on athletes who took creatine for 21 months found no significant changes in markers of kidney function; a 2008 study on athletes who took creatine for 3 months found no evidence of kidney damage during that time. A review found creatine to have no effects on liver of kidney function in over months of supplementation in both young and old population. However, authors still cautioned against using high doses(>3g-5g) in those with impaired kidney function and suggested further studies are needed relating to claims of mutagenicity and carcinogenicity. Other research has shown that oral creatine supplementation at a rate of five to 20 grams per day appears to be very safe and largely devoid of adverse side-effects, while at the same time effectively improving the physiological response to resistance exercise, increasing the maximal force production of muscles in both men and women.

Nevertheless, while some research indicates that supplementation with pure creatine is safe, commercially available supplements can contain potentially harmful contaminants.

Dehydroepiandrosterone (DHEA) is a hormone produced by the adrenal glands. It is also made in the brain. DHEA is implicated in the production of male and female sex hormones, androgens and estrogens. After age 30, DHEA levels in the body begin to decrease, as part of the normal aging process. Lower DHEA levels are also found in people with hormonal disorders, HIV/AIDS, Alzheimer's disease, heart disease, depression, diabetes, inflammation, immune disorders, and osteoporosis. Prescription drugs can also also reduce DHEA levels, such as corticosteroids, birth control pills and medications used to treat psychiatric disorders.

Some data suggests that DHEA may help in the treatment of depression, obesity, hormonal disorders and osteoporosis, but more research is needed to support these findings, as DHEA may cause a number of undesirable side effects. Specifically, women may develop oily skin, a deeper voice, irregular periods, smaller breast size, increased size of the clitoris and increased hair. Men may develop breast tenderness, reduced size of the testes and urinary symptoms, irritability and aggression. Other side effects that may affect both, men and women, include acne, sleep problems, headache, nausea, skin itching, and mood changes. DHEA may also affect levels of other hormones, insulin, and cholesterol and may increase the risk of prostate, breast, and ovarian cancers.

Although DHEA is currently being used by many athletes, there are no published studies on the effect of DHEA on athletic performance.(http://www.wellness. com/reference/herb/dhea)

"Anabolic steroids" is the familiar name for synthetic substances related to the male sex hormones (e.g., testosterone). They promote the growth of skeletal muscle (anabolic effects) and the development of male sexual characteristics (androgenic effects) in both males and females. Anabolic steroids are derivatives of testosterone. The primary medical uses of these compounds are to treat delayed puberty, some types of impotence, and wasting of the body caused by HIV infection or other diseases.

During the 1930s, scientists discovered that anabolic steroids could facilitate the growth of skeletal muscle in laboratory animals, which led to abuse of the compounds first by bodybuilders and weightlifters and then by athletes in other sports. Steroid abuse has become so widespread in athletics that it can affect the outcome of sports contests. These drugs are used to enhance athletic performance, as they promote growth of skeletal muscle and may increase lean body mass. The use of anabolic steroids is illegal without a prescription, The purchase of these supplements, with the notable exception of dehydroepiandrosterone (DHEA), became illegal after the passage in 2004 of amendments to the Controlled Substances Act. Illicit steroids are often sold at gyms, competitions, and through mail order operations after being smuggled into this country. Most illegal steroids in the United States are smuggled from countries that do not require a prescription for the purchase of steroids. Steroids are also illegally diverted from U.S. pharmacies or synthesized in clandestine laboratories. Anabolic steroids have many adverse effects. These include shrinkage of both testicles and penis with decrease in sperm count, masculinization in women with development of excessive body hair, early maturation of the body's long bones with consequent reduction in height. Steroids can also cause decreased glucose tolerance, worsened lipid profile and accelerated hardening of the arteries leading to higher risk for early heart disease. Other side effects include acne and hair loss from the scalp. Mood swings, personality changes, aggression and irritability may occur. There is also a correlation with malignancies and sudden cardiac death.

In addition to increasing muscle mass and improving athletic performance, some adolescents abuse steroids as part of a pattern of high-risk behaviors. These adolescents also take risks such as drinking and driving, carrying a gun, driving a motorcycle without a helmet, and abusing other illicit drugs. Conditions such as muscle dysmorphia, a history of physical or sexual abuse, or a history of engaging in high-risk behaviors have all been associated with an increased risk of initiating or continuing steroid abuse. (https://www.drugabuse.gov/publications/research-reports/anabolic-steroid-abuse/what-are-anabolic-steroids)

Part II

Common Symptoms
and Important Medical
Conditions in Adolescents

Useful on line resources for the medical conditions discussed in part II of the book include the Mayo Clinic website (www.mayoclinic.org), Medical News Today (www.medicalnewstoday.com), Medicine Net (www.medicinenet.com), Wikipedia (www.wikipedia.org), the American Mental Wellness Association (www.americanmentalwellness.org), Mental Health.gov (www.mentalhealth.gov) and others as well, which are mentioned in the pertinent chapters.

Fatigue

Fatigue, a decreased energy level, is one of the most common complaints, not only of adult patients but also of young people. It is necessary to differentiate a significant medical problem from symptoms due to poor sleep habits, alcohol intake, deconditioning, lack of exercise, and an unbalanced diet. In other words, we need to distinguish a pathologic process from an unhealthy life style. You know that if you party too hard, sleep very little, drink alcohol and smoke, you will feel rotten. There are situations, however, when you need to call your doctor for a medical evaluation since numerous illnesses can cause fatigue and lack of energy.

Iron deficiency anemia is a common condition in young women. The body needs sufficient iron to produce red blood cells. When your red blood cell count is low, you feel tired and have no energy around the clock, not just on Monday mornings or after exercise. The anemia may be caused by the blood lost during the menstrual period. Blood is loaded with iron, so having your period, particularly if it is heavy, is an iron drain. If you do not eat enough iron-rich foods, like red meat, fish, turkey, beans, eggs, rice, enriched grains, and leafy green vegetables, your diet does not replace the lost iron. Your doctor can tell if you are anemic with a blood test and prescribe iron supplements if necessary. The iron tablets will supply your body with extra iron to replenish your red blood cell count. After taking the pills for a few weeks, you should pep right up. One side effect of iron tablets is constipation, so it is advisable to eat more fibers like bran cereal or over-the-counter fiber products and drink lots of water. In two to three months, go back to your doctor so that he/she can test your blood to confirm that the blood count is normal. Although you may no longer need iron tablets, you should eat the iron-rich foods mentioned above to compensate for continuing iron losses.

Thyroid disorders can also make you feel tired. The thyroid is an endocrine gland located in our neck in front of the trachea. This gland produces hormones, which have an essential role in metabolism. If the production of thyroid hormone decreases, our body will slow down, and one of the most prominent symptoms will be fatigue and also depressed mood. An increased production of thyroid hormone can also cause fatigue because it stimulates the metabolism excessively, causing fast heart rate, high blood pressure, weight loss, and anxiety. Your doctor can diagnose a thyroid disorder by requesting specific blood tests. Both types of thyroid disorders can be treated.

One very important metabolic disorder, which is increasing among adolescents, is **diabetes mellitus.** The prominent symptoms are persistent, increased thirst, hunger, and urination associated with weight loss and fatigue. Your physician can make the diagnosis with appropriate blood tests, which reveal elevated blood sugar.

A low energy level can also be caused by infectious diseases such as **mononucleosis.** "Mono" presents with sore throat, swollen glands, fever and fatigue. This is the so-called "kissing" disease but it may be acquired simply through close contact and not necessarily requires kissing. The diagnosis may be confirmed by a specific blood test. Treatment usually involves rest and adequate fluid intake. Antibiotics are not necessary since this is a viral infection, but they may be used if a secondary bacterial infection is found. Even after the infection has resolved, the fatigue may persist for weeks. Fatigue may be associated with a variety of infections, either viral such as influenza (flu) or bacterial such as strep throat but the fatigue does not usually persist as long in these conditions as it does after mononucleosis.

Fatigue can also be a result of **inadequate sleep.** The ongoing loss of even one or two hours of sleep per night results in a sleep deficit that can cause loss of energy, irritability, reduced daytime alertness and impaired thinking. There are recommendations for ensuring a good night's sleep. Caffeine is a powerful stimulant and should not be consumed within six hours of bedtime. Many foods, beverages, and medications contain caffeine and should be avoided. Nicotine is also a stimulant; non-smokers are able to fall asleep more quickly than smokers. Alcohol disrupts sleep by reducing the most restful phases, deep sleep and dream or REM (rapid eye movement) sleep. Physical inactivity may contribute to insomnia. Regular exercise helps eliminate this problem. If you find that you have trouble falling asleep, experts suggest that you avoid reading or watching TV in bed and that you create an environment that is conducive to sleep with no loud noise or bright lights.

Diabetes Mellitus

There are two types of diabetes mellitus. Type 1 diabetes mellitus and Type 2 diabetes mellitus. Type 1 diabetes mellitus is much less common than Type 2 diabetes mellitus, accounting for <10 % of cases. It's caused by an autoimmune attack on the insulin producing cells (β-cells) of the pancreas that results in an insulin deficient state, although a small number of functioning β-cells may be present.

Type 1 diabetes is more common in childhood and adolescence. It's characterized by abrupt onset, with symptoms of profound thirst, large production of urine, weight loss and fatigue. Patients often present with a life-threatening condition called diabetic ketoacidosis and require hospitalization and appropriate medical care to survive.

In patients with diabetes mellitus, frequent monitoring of the blood glucose level is needed throughout the day, using a device called glucometer and special test strips on which a drop of blood is placed. Finger pricks with a lancet are used to obtain the blood sample. Several daily injections of insulin, may be needed to achieve optimal blood glucose control. There are now insulin pumps available that can be used to control the blood sugar without having to self-administer frequent injections. Many factors, such as food intake, activity level and illnesses do affect the daily insulin requirement. Therefore, close monitoring is necessary to maintain the blood glucose within a reasonable range and avoid the dangers associated with a glucose that is too high (hyperglycemia) or too low (hypoglycemia). Education by health care personnel is critical to help the newly diagnosed patients to learn about this disease process and its management and to adjust to the demands placed on them by this illness.

Type 2 diabetes is the most common form of the disease, accounting for approximately 90 % of cases. It has a multifactorial disease with a strong genetic component, amplified by factors such as obesity, diet, physical activity, age and pregnancy. Type 2 diabetes is characterized by insufficient secretion of insulin from the β-cells of the pancreas, associated with insulin resistance, which is impaired insulin action in the target tissues such as muscle, liver and fat. Insulin resistance is increased in obesity, which explains why weight gain is associated with a higher risk of Type 2 diabetes.

Type 2 diabetes mellitus was once considered a disease of older adults, but the prevalence of the disease is now progressively increasing in adolescents and younger adults. An inverse relationship exists between body mass index (BMI) and the age of onset of T2DM, which means that the higher the BMI, the lower the age of onset of the disease.

The impact of early onset Type 2 diabetes is significant. The affected individuals are likely to be obese, lead a sedentary lifestyle, have a strong family history of Type

2 diabetes, be of black or minority origin and come from a socially underprivileged group. They have an increased risk of premature development of vascular complications, in addition to psychological morbidity, during their life.

Type 2 diabetes can be treated with weight loss, through adequate diet and exercise, in addition to oral drugs and insulin. The American Diabetes Association, http://www.diabetes.org, offers a wealth of information on the care and treatment of DM and life style changes that are critical in the management of this disease.

Hypertension

High blood pressure, known as hypertension, is a common medical condition in which the force of the blood against the artery walls is high and, if left untreated for a long time, it can cause serious health problems, such as heart disease and stroke. Headaches, shortness of breath, fatigue, chest pressure and other aspecific symptoms might be experienced by people with elevated blood pressure, but, even when the blood pressure readings reach dangerously high levels, most people are asymptomatic, which means they have no signs or symptoms. Therefore, it's critical to understand that, even without symptoms, damage of high blood pressure to the blood vessels and the internal organs continues and that's why hypertension is called the silent killer. Uncontrolled high blood pressure can lead to heart attacks and strokes, rupture of a brain aneurysm, heart failure, kidney failure, vision loss, memory loss, dementia, poor circulation. The higher your blood pressure and the longer it goes uncontrolled, the greater the damage.

High blood pressure is more common in adults, but children and younger adults are at risk too, due to increasing obesity, lack of exercise and unhealthy diet.

The risk factors of high blood pressure include family history, tobacco and alcohol use, being overweight or obese, sedentary life style, excessive amount of salt in the diet, in addition to stress, age, race (high blood pressure is particularly common among blacks, often developing at an earlier age than it does in whites) and other factors.

For most adults, there's no specific, identifiable cause of high blood pressure. High blood pressure tends to be familial and is likely determined by the interaction between environmental and genetic factors. This type of high blood pressure is called primary (essential) hypertension.

In some people, high blood pressure may be caused by other underlying medical problems. This type of high blood pressure is called secondary hypertension. Various conditions and medications can lead to secondary hypertension, such as hormonal disregulation, tumors, kidney problems, thyroid problems, obstructive sleep apnea, prescription medications and illegal drugs.

Luckily, high blood pressure can be easily detected and treated. Your blood pressure is taken as part of a routine doctor's appointment. If you don't regularly see your doctor, which we strongly recommend you to do, you may be able to get a free blood pressure screening at a health fair or other locations in your community. You can also find machines in pharmacies that will measure your blood pressure for free. Public blood pressure machines, may provide helpful information about your blood pressure, but they may have some limitations, as their accuracy is not guaranteed.

(http://nursestudy.net/2014/12/05/high-blood-pressure-pathophysiology/

http://www.mayoclinic.org/diseases-conditions/high-blood-pressure/basics/risk-factors/con-20019580)

Hypercholesterolemia

Hypercholesterolemia is the presence of high levels of cholesterol in the blood. Although hypercholesterolemia per se does not cause any symptoms, it's a major risk factor for atherosclerosis, which leads to hardening of arteries and progressive narrowing of the arterial lumen, due to plaque formation. These plaques form over a long period of time and may slowly lead to complete obstruction of the blood flow. However, a plaque rupture will cause a clot to form and obstruct blood flow abruptly. If this happens in a coronary artery, it may cause a heart attack, while blockage of a brain artery can cause a stroke.

Hypercholesterolemia is typically due to a combination of genetic factors and environmental factors, such as obesity, poor diet, alcohol consumption and sedentary life style.

A number of medical conditions can also increase cholesterol levels including diabetes mellitus type 2, low thyroid function, and certain hormonal disorders.

Even if he U.S. Preventive Services Task Force in 2016 concluded that testing the general population under the age of 40 without symptoms is of unclear benefit, it is now well documented that there is an increasing number of children and adolescents with elevated cholesterol level, therefore early testing might be of great value, because this condition can lead to narrowed and hardened arteries, increasing the risk of atherosclerotic disease later in life.

The first treatment approach for high cholesterol in younger patients involves lifestyle changes that can benefit the entire family: weight loss, eating healthy foods and exercise.

In particular, avoid processed foods that contain large amounts of saturated fats and sugars; eat fruits, vegetable and grains; be more active throughout the day and minimize the amount of time spent in front of computers, tablets, televisions and phones. The doctor might suggest cholesterol medications if you continue to have high cholesterol despite lifestyle changes; are at least 10 years old; have other health problems, such as diabetes or high blood pressure; have a genetic type of high cholesterol.

(https://www.turkaramamotoru.com/en/ hypercholesterolemia-24553.html)

Depression/ Anxiety/ Stress

Depression is a condition accompanied by a lack of interest in things you previously enjoyed and a persistent sense of sadness or hopelessness. Feeling sad on occasion is a normal part of life but when it becomes overwhelming it can signal a more significant problem. Symptoms of depression may seem contradictory but include sleeping too much or too little (insomnia), over-eating or under-eating (loss of appetite), and a decreased energy level. People who are depressed may also experience unexplained headaches, stomachaches, or backaches. They tend to be less active than previously and lose interest in previously rewarding or enjoyable activities. People suffering from clinical depression lose interest in hobbies, friends, work, even food and sex. They also experience a loss of self-esteem and feelings of worthlessness and inadequacy. The exact cause of depression remains unclear, but certain factors do appear to be involved. Depression may run in families. If members of your family are depressed, it is more likely that you may experience similar symptoms. Victims of abusive behavior, whether physical or verbal, may develop emotional disturbances leading to depression. Alcohol and drug use are well known to cause depressive disorders. If you sense that you are depressed, it is important to consult your doctor and not to ignore this serious problem for fear of embarrassment. Depression can be treated with both medication and counseling. Spending time with supportive friends and family, exercising, or playing with pets may also help you through this difficult time. Depression is often associated with anxiety. Common symptoms of anxiety are air hunger leading to hyperventilation, palpitations, sweating, trembling, and a feeling of 'butterflies' in the stomach. Anxiety may also occur without associated depression. People may normally experience mild symptoms of anxiety during particularly stressful times, such as taking a test, moving to a new city or changing schools or jobs. In some individuals the symptoms of anxiety may become constant and pervasive and affect one's daily life. Panic attacks are an extreme form of anxiety characterized by sudden episodes in which the person feels a sense of terror and of imminent catastrophe for no apparent reason. These episodes may last from a few minutes to one or two hours during which the individual is unable to recognize that there is no objective threat.

A certain amount of stress is unavoidable and can be even stimulating but when stress becomes excessive or chronic, it can take a toll on our body and mind. It may lead to physical symptoms of fatigue, malaise, body aches and exacerbate many illnesses. People who are stressed may feel anxious and overwhelmed. They may not be able to concentrate or think clearly. Often people's reaction to an event rather than the event itself causes them stress. This may be due to individual perceptions and differences in coping skills. We cannot always control or change a situation, but we can adjust the way we respond to it. A network of supportive friends and family members, a healthy lifestyle, physical exercise, and adequate rest will all help to minimize the effects of stress. If you find that you are unable to adapt and cope with your circumstances, then it is important to seek professional help. People who are depressed, anxious, or extremely stressed experience a sense of emotional pain that can be as unpleasant as the pain associated with physical illness or trauma.

Headaches

Most headaches fall into three main categories: muscle tension, migraine, and headaches from other causes. Muscle tension headaches are caused by tension in the muscles of the neck, head, and shoulders. They may result from incorrect posture or awkward body positioning, fatigue, and stress. Typical symptoms are pain over the eyes or at the back of the head and band-like pressure around the head that may spread over the entire head into the back of the neck and shoulders.

Migraine symptoms consist of recurring, throbbing, intense pain that usually, but not always, affects one side of the head. Prior to the onset of the actual headache, many people experience what is referred to as an aura, which may include visual changes such as shimmering or flashing lights, blurred vision, and extreme sensitivity to light (photophobia), nausea, irritability, and restlessness. The symptoms may be so distressing that people prefer to lie quietly in a darkened room. Migraine headaches tend to begin between the age of ten and thirty and tend to run in families. They are more common in women than men. Substances that may trigger migraines in some people include foods such as chocolate, nuts, cheese, citrus fruits, dairy products, pickles, cured meats, and MSG (monosodium glutamate). Certain drugs such as birth control pills may also cause migraine headaches. If the migraine headaches are very frequent, preventive treatment is used to reduce the frequency and severity of attacks. There are now also drugs that are taken at the immediate onset of an aura to block the progression of the migraine headache.

Headaches that do not fall into the two previous categories can have numerous causes ranging from iron deficiency anemia, eye problems, allergies, sinus problems, sleep deprivation, colds and influenza, to more serious conditions such as meningitis and intra-cranial processes including brain tumors and hemorrhage.

Eating Disorders

A number of disorders revolve around the misuse of food. Obesity is the number one nutritional problem in the United States.

Although certain medications (for example anti-depressants, steroids, birth control pills) and hormonal imbalances such as hypothyroidism may cause some weight gain, obesity is a disorder that results from an imbalance between the calories consumed and those burned each day. While there may be a genetic predisposition that makes certain people more prone to gain weight, the diet (portion size and type of food) and a sedentary lifestyle remain significant factors. The prevalence of obesity among children and adolescents is rising at an alarming rate. Excessive weight can have a number of bad effects on your health and how you feel about yourself. Being obese increases your chances of developing diabetes, and not just later in life: several reports show that obesity is associated with the increased incidence in diabetes recently observed in children and teenagers. Being obese also puts you at risk of developing high blood pressure, cardiovascular disease, gall bladder disease, colon cancer, and breast cancer. The added weight places additional stress on the joints and may result in early arthritis, back pain, and knee pain. Significant psychological and emotional distress may develop in overweight adolescents.

There is no magic food, diet pill or activity that can solve the problem of excess weight. Most nutrition professionals favor a combination of eating fewer calories and increasing physical activity. Helpful hints to lose weight include: decreasing portion size, reducing intake of high calorie snacks, not keeping tempting foods around the house, eating slowly with awareness of every bite you eat, eating in only one location in your home, preferably at the dining table, without activities that distract you such as watching television, and keeping food records. Many people who overeat often crave a particular food that has nothing to do with them actually being hungry. Cravings generally fade in less than 30 minutes so find something else to occupy yourself, and the craving may pass. Increased physical activity is the other aspect of any successful weight control plan. Not only does exercise help you lose weight, it helps tone your body so you look better as you lose body fat. Exercise also takes your mind off food. One of the most discouraging things about losing weight is that most people regain the weight they lose and may even gain a few extra pounds. Research has shown that participating in a regular exercise program is the most important thing you can do to keep off the weight you have lost. Losing weight is not an easy task. It requires the realization that a healthful diet is a lifelong endeavor and not a quick fix. One needs continued focus and commitment to avoid returning to old unhealthy habits. Some people find joining a weight loss program helpful. Don't be fooled by promises of effortless weight loss and miracle diets. Your doctor may refer you to a registered dietician for help with a healthful eating program and an exercise professional to help you with a safe and appropriate program of regular physical activity.

At the other end of the spectrum of eating disorders are anorexia, bulimia, and binge eating. These are common and potentially life threatening eating disorders. The National Association of Anorexia Nervosa and Associated Disorders states that approximately eight million people in the U.S. have anorexia nervosa, bulimia, and related eating disorders. Eight million people represents about three percent (3%) of the total population (https://www.anred.com). Anorexia occurs in approximately 1% of American women and is defined as intentional self-starvation leading to weight loss of at least 15% below normal body weight. It often includes compulsive exercise to keep the weight off. Even when anorectic individuals are exceedingly thin, they remain convinced they are overweight, and they have an unreasonable fear of gaining any weight at all. Bulemia occurs in about 1.5% of American women. It involves binging (consuming large amounts of food) followed by purging (getting rid of food by vomiting or by misusing laxatives, diuretics, or enemas). It may be difficult to identify because the binging and purging are done in secret, and bulimic individuals usually maintain a normal body weight. Bulemia may also include excessive exercise. Some people suffer from both anorexia and bulimia and have symptoms of both. Binge eating disorder affects about 2.8% of the general population and is more common in women. It consists of episodes of uncontrolled eating until the individual is uncomfortably full. There are many factors that contribute to the development of an eating disorder. Psychological, social, and cultural issues play a large role in these diseases. Our society associates beauty with being thin. Girls are constant barraged by messages that lead them to identify their self-worth with the attainment of an idealized body image. Pre-teen girls in our society are already aware of this cultural mandate, and many girls are known to attempt diets and other measures to control their weight. Since only a small proportion of adolescents develop this disturbed sense of body image leading to these eating disorders, other causes must be involved such as still undefined psychological or genetic factors. There are serious health consequences to these eating disorders occurs. Amenorrhea is universal in anorectic females, and often appears before appreciable weight loss. In the malnourished anorectic patient, dysfunction may be found in virtually every major organ system, the most dangerous being cardiac and fluid/electrolyte disorders. Sudden death may occur due to ventricular arrhythmias. In bulimics, the induced vomiting is associated with erosion of dental enamel, esophagitis, esophageal rupture, and aspiration pneumonia. Electrolyte abnormalities also may result from vomiting or excessive use of laxatives. Binge eaters typically are overweight, placing them at higher risk for the medical problems associated with obesity. All of these disorders are associated with psychiatric problems, especially depression. Obviously medical intervention is necessary but, unfortunately, a common feature of these disorders is secrecy and denial of the problem. Therefore, these patients commonly do not receive the treatment they need until they present with advanced problems.

Muscle Dysmorphia and Body Dysmorphic Disorder (BDD)

Although eating disorders have been viewed as female issues, anorexia, bulimia, and especially binge-eating disorder are increasingly diagnosed in the male population. Anorexia, for example, is now diagnosed in boys as young as eight and up to 40% of people with binge-eating disorders are males. Several factors contribute to this phenomenon.

Boys are now feeling the pressure to be physically perfect, which, in the past, was directed almost exclusively at girl. Therefore, they are just as likely as girls to develop an unrealistic body image of what a male body should look like: big, muscular, lean and fit, like the various action figures and male models in fashion and advertising. By age 14, boys start to struggle, in various degree, with this ideal body image. The widespread use of anabolic steroids and sport supplements reflects boys' attempts to model their bodies on the idealized images imposed on them by our culture. The danger associated with this process is the development of muscle dysmorphia, a subtype of body dysmorphic disorder (BDD), where the affected individual thinks that his muscles are never big enough; in this condition, the boy is ashamed of muscles he thinks are too small, when, in fact, they are not. They obsess about being undeveloped and the constant preoccupation with perceived smallness eventually interferes with school, social interaction, relationships and career accomplishments.

In body dysmorphic disorder, a normal appearing person believes he or she is physically abnormal or defective, causing severe emotional distress and difficulties in daily functioning. The perceived defect may be only a slight imperfection or nonexistent. People with BDD can dislike any part of their body, although they often find fault with their hair, skin, nose, chest, or stomach. This disorder develops in adolescents and teens, and it affects men and women almost equally A severe form of BDD may cause the individual to become extremely self-conscious and so preoccupied with his/her appearance that he/she will stop seeing friends, drop out of activities and become completely isolated. (https://www.eatingdisorderhope.com/treatment-for-eating-disorders/special-issues/men)

Obsessive-Compulsive Disorder (OCD)

OCD symptoms usually start in adolescence or early adulthood. The prevalence is higher among women and tends to decline with age. The essential features of OCD are recurrent, resisted, troubling thoughts, or obsessions (such as "objects are contaminated") and repetitive but unnecessary actions, or compulsions (such as washing hands or turning off lights over and over again). The most common obsessions are fear of contamination, fear of acting aggressively, and fear of doing something harmful or unacceptable that the individual perceives as totally alien to himself/herself as a person. Such thoughts occur independently of his/her own will and he spends considerable energy trying to resist them but inevitably the ideas return moments later. Compulsions are actions the person takes to try to neutralize the obsessive thoughts through repetitive acts or rituals. Although the person recognizes these urges as absurd, they are generally overwhelming and he/she must comply in order to combat the anxiety generated by the impulse. The most common compulsions involve checking, cleaning, and counting. In most cases, the symptoms are chronic and continuous with a tendency to worsen during stressful times. Other psychiatric disorders may also be associated with OCD such as major depression, phobia, and panic disorder. While the cause of OCD remains unclear, there is some evidence to suggest a higher incidence in identical twins and in the families of OCD patients compared to the general population implying the possible role of both genetic and environmental factors. Treatment of OCD includes both psychotherapy and medications such as tricyclic antidepressants and serotonin uptake inhibitors.

Attention Deficit/Hyperactivity Disorder (ADHD)

The National Survey of Children's Health (NSCH) 2003–2011, based on parent interviews, shows that 5.1 million children age 4-17 (8.8% or 1 in 11 of this age group 4–17 years) have a current diagnosis of ADHD.

Attention-deficit/hyperactivity disorder (ADHD) is a brain disorder characterized by inattention and/or hyperactivity-impulsivity that interferes with functioning or development.

Inattention means a person has difficulty sustaining focus and is disorganized. Symptoms of inattention include failure to follow through on instructions, failure to complete school work or duties, easy distractibility, avoidance of tasks that require sustained effort, and difficulty organizing activities.

Hyperactivity means a person has a need to move constantly, including when is not appropriate. Symptoms of hyperactivity include inability to remain seated, squirming, running, difficulty awaiting one's turn, talking and fidgeting excessively.

Impulsivity means a person makes hasty decisions without thinking about possible harmful consequences, tendency to blurt out answers before a question is completed and to interrupt or intrude into conversations or games.

Multiple symptoms of either inattention or hyperactivity/impulsivity must be present in order to make the diagnosis of ADHD. Most children with ADHD are diagnosed during the elementary school years. The diagnosis requires a comprehensive evaluation by health care professionals, such as a pediatrician, psychologist, or psychiatrist with expertise in ADHD.

ADHD symptoms can appear as early as between the ages of 3 and 6 and can continue through adolescence and adulthood. Symptoms of ADHD can be missed, leading to a delay in diagnosis. Many adolescents and adults with ADHD struggle with academic performance, work performance, have difficulties with relationships and may display antisocial behaviors.

Medications as well as psychotherapy, family therapy, behavior modification programs, and support groups play a pivotal role in the reatment of ADHD. The medications target and stimulate the areas of the brain specifically involved with attention. Some children require long-term use of stimulant drugs through high school and college. Through behavioral therapy, they can be guided to devote their extra energy to school projects, sports activities and hobbies, and they may become successful in many areas.

(https://www.nimh.nih.gov)

(http://www.psychiatricholistichealth.com/ADHDADD.en.html)

Seizure Disorders

A seizure is a spontaneous, transient burst of abnormal electrical brain activity that results in the sudden onset of altered consciousness, motor activity, sensory phenomena, or inappropriate behavior.

Convulsive seizures are the most common form of attacks and may be partial or generalized. Partial seizures are characterized by involuntary movements of the head and arms with or without loss of contact with the surroundings and with or without other sensory manifestations. Generalized seizures are characterized by sudden loss of consciousness with muscular contractions and rigidity of the entire body. Absence attacks are generalized seizures in which the patient suddenly stops any activity in which he/she is engaged and is oblivious to the surroundings for 10-30 seconds. These absence seizures start before the age of twenty. They may occur several times a day often while the person is sitting quietly. Approximately 2.5 to 3 million people in the U.S. have epilepsy. The incidence is highest in children and adolescents. There are numerous medications available for treatment. Some patients require lifetime treatment and medical supervision.

Seizures also can be caused by congenital brain lesions that are present since birth, head trauma, brain tumors, infections such as meningitis and encephalitis, and high fever. Metabolic disorders such as hypoglycemia, hyperglycemia, hyponatremia, and hypocalcemia can cause seizures as well. Drug use and drug withdrawal can both cause seizures. Cocaine use may induce convulsions and delirium. Alcohol withdrawal may result in seizures and altered mental status as well. Acute convulsions from febrile illnesses, alcohol withdrawal, drug toxicity, and metabolic disturbances require emergency treatment for both the causative condition as well as for the convulsion.

Since a seizure may occur anywhere, it is useful to be familiar with the appropriate method of handling a convulsing patient. If the patient has lost consciousness, ease them to the ground and turn the head to one side to protect them from aspirating their own saliva or vomit. Although in the past people have been told to put something in the patient's mouth to prevent tongue biting, this action can cause further injury and is not advisable.

Allergies

The most common form of allergy is allergic rhinitis which includes both seasonal rhinitis (hay fever) and perennial rhinitis (yearlong). Symptoms include itchy, watery eyes, sneezing, runny or stuffy nose, post-nasal drip, headache and fatigue. Allergy symptoms may be similar to cold symptoms but usually last longer and may worsen during spring or fall.

Allergies seem to run in families. Hay fever usually develops in childhood but can occur at any age. Allergies that occur in spring and fall are due to tree, grass, or weed pollen. Allergies that persist all year long may be due to dust mites, mold spores, or animal dander. The most common indoor allergens are house dust, cockroaches, and dust mites. Antihistamine medication and nasal corticosteroid spray help to reduce nasal congestion and other symptoms by blocking the allergic response. With perennial allergies, avoidance of exposure to household dust or animal dander is key to the management of the disease. More severe cases may require desensitization, which is a process of using repeated injections of the triggering materials to block the allergic response.

Some people have allergies to insect stings, certain foods or medications. Examples include bee stings, nuts, peanuts which are responsible for very severe food induced allergic reactions, shellfish, penicillin and sulfa drugs. The allergic reaction may range from a generalized skin rash with itching to a more severe and life-threatening condition in which the person becomes flushed and agitated, and complains of palpitations, itching, and trouble breathing. Without immediate intervention the person may soon become unresponsive and die (anaphylactic shock). If you have had a severe allergic reaction, doctors suggest that you carry an epinephrine syringe designed for self-administration to decrease the severity of the reaction until further medical care becomes available. A medical identification bracelet should be worn if you have experienced significant allergic reactions. This will alert people in the event that you are unresponsive.

Swimmer's Ear

Otitis externa is an inflammation or infection of the external auditory canal the auricle, or both. This condition can be found in all age groups and presents with pain, ear fullness, decreased hearing, tinnitus (ringing in the ear), itching and discharge.

Swimmer's ear is a bacterial infection of the external ear canal that can develops after water has gotten in the ear, especially after swimming. Sand or other debris that get into the ear canal may also cause swimmer's ear. Symptoms include pain, itching and a feeling of fullness in the ear. The ear canal may become swollen and red. A discharge may be present and there may be some hearing loss. In order to avoid this problem, it is important to keep the ears dry. Using cotton swabs, however, may irritate the canal. It is best, therefore, to tilt the head from side to side and gently to dry your ears using a tissue or towel. Using a few drops of rubbing alcohol in each ear after swimming may help; but should not be used if there is a perforation of the eardrums. If symptoms of an infection develop, your primary care physician can prescribe eardrops, which will usually clear the infection in one week.

Fungal Infections

Fungal infection of the skin most commonly affects the feet, groin, scalp and nails. Fungi grow best in warm, moist areas of the skin such a between the toes, in the groin, and in the area beneath the breasts. Athlete's foot (tinea pedis) is the most common fungal skin infection. Symptoms include redness, peeling, and itching between the toes and on the soles.

The skin may also weep or ooze clear or yellowish fluid. This condition often recurs and must be treated each time. Jock itch (tinea cruris) causes similar symptoms in the groin and upper thighs. Fungal infections of the fingernails or toenails (onychomycosis) are more common in adults. They cause discoloration and thickening of the nails and may be difficult to treat. To prevent fungal infections of the skin, it is important to keep these areas cool and dry. Drying off well, especially after exercise, applying talcum powder to the feet, groin, and under the breasts, and wearing socks that wick away moisture are useful measures. Even though there are antifungal products available over-the-counter, we recommend seeking medical advice to assure appropriate treatment.

Lymph Nodes

The lymph nodes are small glands found throughout the body that may become noticeable in the neck, the axillae, and the groin. The lymph nodes swell in response to infections or insect bites. Swelling in the glands on either side of the neck may occur with throat infections.

Swelling in the glands in the back of the neck may be due to scalp conditions. Cat-scratch disease is a bacterial infection acquired from even minor cat scratches and most commonly from kittens. Lymph nodes will swell in specific areas in relation to the scratch site. For example, if the scratch is on the hand or arm, the axillary (underarm) lymph nodes or the nodes at the elbow may swell. If the scratch is on the foot or leg, the inguinal (groin) lymph nodes will be affected. Enlargement of the inguinal lymph nodes may be due to sexually transmitted diseases. There are also very serious conditions such as leukemia and other types of cancer that can cause swelling of the lymph nodes. Swollen lymph nodes, whether tender or painless, should be evaluated by a physician.

Sudden Cardiac Death

Sudden death in a young person is a rare, devastating event defined as death that is abrupt, unexpected, and due to a cardiovascular cause. It is generally recognized as death that occurs within 1 hour from the onset of cardiovascular symptoms. However, in young people, it typically occurs within a few minutes of symptom onset. Sports participation has been associated with an increased risk of SCD in young people. Therefore, cardiovascular screening for conditions that could lead to an increased risk of sudden death is recommended prior to enrolling in sport activities. In the United States, current recommendations include a focused personal and family history of the athlete with special emphasis on history of exertional chest pain, syncope or a family history of early sudden death, as well as examination for blood pressure, murmurs, and stigmata of Marfan's syndrome. If any abnormalities are found, additional studies are initiated to systematically exclude known causes of sudden death.

Most causes of sudden cardiac death in young people are due to heart abnormalities that may have been asymptomatic and therefore unrecognized. The most common of these are hypertrophic cardiomyopathy, left ventricular hypertrophy, dilated cardiomyopathy and congenital coronary artery anomalies. There are some less common causes of sudden cardiac death, which include abnormalities of the heart valves and rhythm disturbances, which may lead to electrical instability that leads to a fatal arrhythmia. Coronary artery disease in adolescents, unlike in the adult population, is an unlikely cause of sudden death. When we say coronary artery disease, we refer to atherosclerotic blockages in the coronary arteries, and adolescents are too young to have developed significant blockages.

Drugs such as cocaine and anabolic steroids have been associated with sudden cardiac death. Cocaine can trigger a spasm of the coronary arteries leading to massive heart attacks even in young people. Anabolic steroids, by producing hypertension and increasing the cholesterol levels, increase cardiovascular risk. Sudden death in patients with anorexia nervosa and bulimia may be due to electrolyte abnormalities causing cardiac arrest.

Prior to engaging in significant physical activity, it is best to consult your physician who will review your medical and family history. Dizziness, light-headedness, or loss of consciousness may indicate underlying heart problems such as hypertrophic cardiomyopathy, arrhythmias, or valvular problems. Chest pain during or after exercise may indicate coronary artery anomalies or other types of cardiovascular disease. Shortness of breath out of proportion to physical activity may suggest heart or lung disease. Palpitations may signal arrhythmias and conduction abnormalities. The presence of a heart murmur may raise some concerns although in the vast majority of cases the murmurs detected in adolescents are benign. A family history of sudden death before the age of fifty is extremely important because some causes of death can be familial and this should stimulate more in-depth cardiac evaluation. It is also important to discuss any drug use with your physician; this includes alcohol, tobacco, cocaine, and other illegal drugs, anabolic steroids, and sports supplements. Cardiopulmonary resuscitation (CPR) classes have traditionally been available to adults. More recently adolescents have been encouraged to participate in CPR training since they too may witness a cardiac event and be available to assist in resuscitation before emergency personnel arrive.

Respiratory Infections

Respiratory problems can be as simple as a minor cold or as life-threatening as an asthma attack or pneumonia. The 'common cold' is caused by many different viruses. Symptoms include runny nose, sneezing, sinus congestion, sore throat, headache, and malaise. It may also involve the larynx or voice box and cause hoarseness. There is a gradual one or two day onset of symptoms that may last up to two weeks. Colds occur throughout the year but are most common in late winter and early spring. There is currently no cure for the common cold. The virus is transmitted by air-borne particles or by contact with contaminated surfaces. Therefore, it is important to avoid close contact and shared utensils or towels with people who have a cold. Home treatment of a cold will help relieve symptoms. It is not necessary to stay in bed, but it is recommended to rest as much as possible and drink lots of fluids. You can use over-the-counter medication such as decongestants, antihistamines and pain relievers to help with the many different symptoms. It is common to have moderately swollen and painful tonsils with a cold. The tonsils are lymphatic tissues in the throat that help fight infections by the production of antibodies. Tonsillitis, inflammation of the tonsils, refers to infection of the tonsils from viruses or streptococcal bacteria. High fever, swollen lymph nodes in the neck, malaise, headache and occasionally abdominal pain, vomiting and diarrhea may accompany tonsillitis. The sore throat and pain is most marked on swallowing and may even cause earache. Streptococcal tonsillitis or 'strep throat' must be treated with antibiotics in order to prevent the complication of rheumatic fever, a severe illness which affects the heart, joints, skin, and nerves. Another cause of sore throat, besides the common cold, is infectious mononucleosis, which is due to the Epstain-Barr virus. In addition to severe sore throat, fever, and swollen lymph nodes in the neck, symptoms of 'mono' include persistent fatigue and body aches. These symptoms may last for several weeks to months. There is no specific medical treatment other than rest and fluids. Your doctor will establish the proper diagnosis and treatment.

Sinusitis is an inflammation or infection of the sinuses, hollow cavities within the bones of the face. Sinusitis may follow a common cold and is usually caused by bacteria. Symptoms include fever, pain in the cheek bones, upper teeth, or forehead and thick, greenish-brown mucous from the nose or down the back of the throat. Antibiotics are used to treat the infection.

Coughing is the body's way of removing foreign material or mucous from the lungs. A dry, or nonproductive, cough does not produce sputum and may develop towards the end of a cold or after exposure to an irritant such as dust or smoke. A dry cough may follow viral respiratory illnesses, may last up to several weeks and is often worse at night. A productive cough is accompanied by a feeling of congestion in the chest and production of mucous from the lungs. The mucous is usually thick and yellowish-green and will clear as the infection resolves. A productive cough can be a symptom of bronchitis or pneumonia. Bronchitis refers to infection of the bronchial tubes, and pneumonia refers to infection of the lung tissue. Both can be caused by viruses or bacteria. Symptoms of bacterial pneumonia include fever, shaking chills, shortness of breath, pain in the chest wall with cough or a deep breath, and production of thick, yellow-green sputum. Some microorganisms (atypical bacteria) can cause a less severe type of pneumonia, called 'walking pneumonia', in which the affected person is generally still able to be relatively active,. Antibiotics are needed for the treatment of bacterial bronchitis and pneumonia.

A persistent dry cough may be a symptom of asthma. Asthma is a condition that causes obstruction of the airways. The muscle surrounding the bronchial tubes goes into spasm making breathing difficult. Many things can trigger asthma including dust, pollen, mold, and animal dander, exercise, cold air, cigarette smoke, changes in weather, chemical fumes, analgesics such as aspirin, and food preservatives. Respiratory infections may exacerbate asthma and precipitate an asthma attack. During the attack the affected individual develops chest tightness, shortness of breath, wheezing, and cough. This is a serious medical condition that requires immediate medical attention and treatment to avoid potentially fatal outcomes. For effective treatment of asthma it is necessary to avoid exposure to recognized triggers and follow the daily treatment plan outlined by the physician.

Influenza or 'flu' is a viral illness that commonly occurs in the winter and affects many people at once. Symptoms of influenza are similar to those of a cold but develop suddenly and are more severe. They include fever, chills, body aches, headaches, fatigue, runny nose, sore throat and dry cough. Although a person with the flu feels very sick, the illness is potentially dangerous only in infants, the elderly and people with chronic diseases who may develop complications such as life-threatening pneumonia. A vaccine is prepared yearly to protect against the expected strains of the influenza virus. New medications are now available which, if taken early in the course, may reduce the severity of symptoms. Treatment includes the usual remedies of rest, fluid intake, and over-the-counter medications, unless these are contraindicated.

Abdominal Problems

The cause of abdominal problems can be difficult to pin point. Many abdominal problems are minor and respond to home treatment; however, some conditions require prompt evaluation and medical treatment. Symptoms of heartburn, nausea, bloating, diarrhea, constipation, and pain can range from mild to severe. Even mild symptoms that persist can represent a problem. Severe symptoms that occur abruptly, increase over several hours, and are accompanied by fever and chills need immediate attention.

Gastritis is an inflammatory process of the stomach lining which can have many different causes including significant stress, use of aspirin-like products, alcohol intake, viral infections, and a bacteria called Helicobacter Pylori. A person feels a sense of burning discomfort or pain (heartburn) in the upper abdomen and may have some nausea, vomiting, or bloating. Heartburn may occur when stomach acid backs into the lower esophagus, the tube connecting the mouth to the stomach. The medical term for heartburn is gastro-esophageal reflux disease (GERD). The acids produce a burning sensation behind the breastbone or sternum and occasionally a bitter taste in the mouth. Heartburn may be caused by overeating, eating certain foods such as chocolate, citrus fruit, tomatoes, peppermint, caffeine or carbonated drinks, smoking cigarettes and drinking alcohol. People who are overweight have a tendency to experience heartburn. Similar and more severe symptoms may indicate deeper damage in the lining of the stomach (gastric ulcer) or of the upper portion of the small intestine (duodenal ulcer). Ulcers may bleed, causing a person to vomit blood or pass dark black stools. This is a medical emergency requiring immediate intervention.

Gastroenteritis is a group of diseases characterized by nausea, vomiting, diarrhea of variable severity, and abdominal discomfort. It may be caused by an infection with viruses, bacteria, or parasites, or by the toxins produced by certain bacteria (food poisoning). Viral gastroenteritis is a common viral infection of the gastrointestinal system that usually resolves in a few days. It is important to avoid dehydration from watery diarrhea by drinking plenty of liquids. Food poisoning is caused by toxins produced by bacteria grown in improperly handled, stored, or cooked food. The symptoms may begin within a few hours or as long as 48 hours after eating. One common cause of food poisoning is Staphylococcus aureus which can contaminate foods such as custards, cream-filled pastry, milk, fish, and processed meat left at room temperature. Another and potentially more serious cause of food poisoning is Escherichia coli (E. coli). It can occur in isolated cases or in outbreaks from eating undercooked beef or unpasteurized milk. Gastroenteritis can also be caused by other bacteria such as Salmonella and Shigella. Salmonella is found in contaminated foods, mainly poultry, eggs, and meat. Shigella is spread through contaminated food and water and is mainly due to inadequate hand washing. The most common cause of parasitic infection of the intestine is Giardia Lamblia. Giardiasis is a disease acquired by drinking water contaminated by the protozoa. While it occurs worldwide and in many underdeveloped countries, it is actually one of the most common intestinal infections in the U.S.A. Symptoms are commonly mild with intermittent nausea, bloating, upper abdominal pain, bulky stools and occasionally diarrhea. If symptoms of gastroenteritis persist, medical evaluation is required to establish the diagnosis and proper treatment.

Abdominal cramps, nausea, diarrhea and bloating can be caused by inability to digest carbohydrates due to a lack of intestinal enzymes. The most common example is lactose intolerance due to lactase deficiency. Lactose is a carbohydrate present in milk and dairy products. Lactase is the enzyme in the intestinal wall that breaks down lactose into smaller sugars that may then be absorbed. With lactase deficiency undigested lactose remains in the intestine causing diarrhea and bloating. This enzyme deficiency is very common among Orientals, Blacks, and Indians. The disorder is controlled by a lactose free diet, either by avoiding milk and dairy products or by taking Lactaid tablets which will allow the digestion of lactose.

Crohn's disease is an inflammatory process primarily involving the ileum, a portion of the small intestine, and the colon, or large intestine. The cause of this disease is unknown. Most cases begin before the age of thirty with the peak incidence between the ages of fourteen and twenty-four. Symptoms include chronic diarrhea, abdominal pain, fever, anorexia (loss of appetite), and weight loss. This disease may also involve the joints, back, eyes, and kidneys. Ulcerative colitis is another inflammatory process involving the large intestine causing abdominal cramps and bloody diarrhea. It most commonly occurs between the ages of fifteen and thirty. The onset of these diseases can be gradual or sudden. They are both serious conditions requiring long-term treatment.

The appendix is a small sac extending from the large intestine. If it's opening becomes blocked, bacteria can grow, and the appendix may become infected. This condition is known as appendicitis. Appendicitis is most common between the ages of ten and thirty. In most people the appendix lies in the right, lower part of the abdomen. The pain may predominate in that area, but it may also be felt around the belly button or in the entire abdomen. Nausea, vomiting, and fever may also be present. Appendicitis requires surgery. If intervention is delayed, the appendix may rupture and the infection may spread throughout the abdomen leading to a much more serious problem.

Constipation is defined as difficult or infrequent passage of stools. Most people pass stools normally from three times a day to three times a week. These differences may be related to diet, exercise, fluid intake, or a familial trait. For some people adequate and unhurried time may be necessary to allow for passage of stool. Constipation may be accompanied by abdominal cramping and discomfort in the rectum. There may be some bloating and nausea. Occasionally a small amount of bright red blood may be noticed on the stools or tissue if passage of hard stools causes minor tearing of the lining of the rectum or bleeding from hemorrhoids. To prevent constipation it is helpful to eat high fiber foods such as fruits, vegetables, and whole grains, drink plenty of water every day, and exercise regularly.

Hemorrhoids are an enlargement of the veins in the rectal area. Constipation and straining may cause these veins to become enlarged and inflamed. The symptoms of hemorrhoids are pain, itching, and occasionally bleeding. They may feel like a lump around the anus. To prevent hemorrhoids and to keep them from worsening it is important to keep the stools soft. Some over the counter preparations may also help with the symptoms of discomfort and itching.

Irritable bowel syndrome is a common problem of the digestive tract with no known cause and no serious consequences. Symptoms include abdominal pain, bloating, and irregular bowel habits with constipation, diarrhea or both. The symptoms may be triggered by stress or ingestion of certain foods and drinks such as alcohol, caffeine, beans, broccoli, apples, spicy foods, citrus fruits, and fatty foods. Identifying particular triggers may help to avoid or minimize the attacks. If your bowel habits are irregular you should consult your doctor for further evaluation and treatment.

A hernia occurs when the intestines bulge through a weak spot in the abdominal wall. They commonly occur in the groin and in the scrotum in men. Hernias are often caused by increased abdominal pressure resulting from lifting heavy weights, coughing, or straining during bowel movements. Sometimes a weak spot in the abdominal wall is present at birth. Therefore, young children or teenagers may also develop hernias. The main symptom is the bulge sometimes accompanied by a mild discomfort. If the hernia becomes trapped outside the abdominal wall, rapidly increasing pain will develop. This is an emergency requiring immediate medical evaluation and surgical intervention. If you suspect you have a hernia, you should see your doctor.

Reproductive Cycle in Women

The possibility of bear children is due to a complex reproductive system that goes through several phases during a woman's lifespan. In the U.S., girls normally reach menarche, the first menstruation, after age nine and before age sixteen and, typically, between age eleven and fourteen. Each woman is born with about two million undeveloped eggs in her two ovaries. Between three and twelve months after reaching menarche, a girl will begin to ovulate each month, releasing a mature egg from one of the ovaries. From this time, she is capable of becoming pregnant. Although the average menstrual cycle is twenty-eight days, the length can vary from twenty-four to thirty-five days depending on the individual woman. A woman may become pregnant anytime during the menstrual cycle, but the most likely time is around ovulation that occurs about day fourteen from the beginning of the menstrual cycle. Some girls and women may experience pain at the time of ovulation. Most experience mild or intense pain during menstruation consisting of cramps in the lower abdomen and lower back. The pain may be accompanied by headache, fatigue, and in some cases, by nausea, vomiting, dizziness, and a sense of malaise. Pre-menstrual syndrome (PMS) refers to a wide range of physical and emotional symptoms including breast swelling and tenderness, weight gain and bloating, food craving especially for sweets, and mood swings with emotional changes such as crying, anxiety, irritability, and insomnia. PMS occurs in approximately 20% to 30% of women in the one or two weeks preceding their period. The exact cause of PMS remains unknown, but hormonal variations likely play a role. The most effective ways to handle these symptoms include getting sufficient sleep, limiting salt, alcohol and caffeine intake, performing regular exercise, and using the commonly available over-the-counter anti-inflammatory pain medications. Premenstrual dysphoric disorder (PMDD) is a more severe form of PMS that has greater psychological symptoms. PMDD affects three to eight percent of pre-menopausal women and may require the use of antidepressants.

If you choose to use vaginal tampons, they should be left in place for no more than eight hours to avoid toxic-shock syndrome (TSS). This is a syndrome characterized by high fever, vomiting, confusion, and skin rash that may rapidly progress to severe shock. It is caused by a toxin produced by a particular strain of staphylococcus aureus, a bacterium found in various parts of the body. In menstruating women it has been found in the vagina and in almost every case of TSS, the affected women used tampons for their menses. Menstrual cycles that are longer or shorter than the usual twenty-eight days may occur normally in some women. The absence of menstruation, either lack of menarche or cessation of menses, is called amenorrhea. One of the most common causes of amenorrhea is pregnancy. Several other conditions, however, may disrupt the periods including excessive dieting and weight loss, eating disorders, excessive exercise, severe stress, and hormonal disorders. Missing three periods is a generally recommended indication for evaluation by a medical professional. If you have engaged in sexual intercourse, however, you are advised to seek medical assistance at the first missed cycle to determine as soon as possible whether you are pregnant so that you can receive early pre-natal care.

Hormonal stimulation of the breast tissue during the menstrual cycle causes swelling of the blood vessels, enlargement of the milk glands and ducts, and fluid retention, making the breasts feel swollen and painful. This generally resolves at the end of the cycle, which is why self-examination of the breasts is best performed right after the menstrual period. Breast tenderness, however, can also be caused by fibrocystic disease, a condition in which the breast tissue feels more firm and 'lumpy' due to the presence of fluid-filled cysts that may form in obstructed or enlarged milk ducts. Fibrocystic tissue may also feel like tiny beads scattered throughout the breast, particularly in the upper outer quadrant of the breasts. Treatment includes using the commonly available over-the-counter pain relievers, avoidance of caffeine to reduce fluid retention, and wearing a well-fitted support bra.

Vaginitis

Vaginitis is a general term for irritation of the vagina which may be caused by inflammation and/or infection. Vaginitis is a very common problem characterized not only by irritation or local redness but also by itching, burning, and possibly the presence of a discharge. There are several different types of vaginal infections, the most common being bacterial vaginosis, yeast infections, and sexually transmitted diseases.

Bacterial vaginosis is a very common type of vaginal infection caused by an increase in the amount of certain bacteria in the vagina. Although it is not sexually transmitted from partner to partner, it is more common in women who are sexually active. Symptoms of bacterial vaginosis include discharge of clear or yellowish mucous with an unpleasant "fishy" odor. Treatment may include applying an antibiotic cream to the vagina or taking antibiotics.

Yeast infections are characterized by intense itching and burning with redness of the vaginal area and the presence of a white discharge that has the appearance of "cottage cheese". The most common yeast infection is caused by Candida which is normally present in the vagina but may overgrow in certain situations such as diabetes, obesity, taking antibiotics, and pregnancy. Once a yeast infection has been diagnosed it can be treated with vaginal creams or oral medications.

Sexually Transmitted Diseases

Sexually transmitted diseases (STD) are infectious diseases of the genital tract transmitted from partner to partner during sexual intercourse. STDs are very common in both men and women. They can potentially have serious consequences for women. Pelvic inflammatory disease (PID) occurs when the infection spreads from the vaginal area to the fallopian tubes and throughout the pelvic area. PID may be treated but it may cause a chronic inflammatory process leading to abdominal pain, low grade fever, and infertility.

Chlamydia is the most commonly reported STD in the U.S. It's spread mostly by vaginal or anal sex, but you can get it through oral sex, too. Sometimes you'll notice an odd discharge from your vagina or penis, or pain or burning when you pee. Only about 25% of women and 50% of men get symptoms. Chlamydia is caused by bacteria, so it's treated with antibiotics. After you are treated, you should get retested in three months, even if your partner has been treated as well. Chlamydia can cause PID.

Gonorrhea is another common bacterial STD. People often get it with chlamydia, and the symptoms are similar: unusual discharge from the vagina or penis, or pain or burning when you pee. Most men with gonorrhea get symptoms, but only about 20% of women do, allowing the infection to spread to the pelvic female organs and cause PID. Gonorrhea is easily treated with antibiotics. If left untreated, the gonococcus may spread into the blood stream and possibly infect the joints causing pain, swelling, and fever.

More women than men get Trichomonas Vaginalis, which is a parasite. Men and women can give it to each other through penis-vagina contact. Women can give it to each other when their genital areas touch. Only about 30% of people with trichomoniasis have symptoms including itching, burning, or sore genitals. You might also see a smelly, clear, white, yellowish, or greenish discharge. Trichomoniasis is treated with antibiotics. It is important to be retested within three months of treatment, even if your partner has been treated as well.

Syphilis is a bacterial STD that is potentially life threatening. In addition to being transmitted sexually, syphilis can also be transmitted through contact with syphilitic sores on the body of an infected person. In the initial stage of syphilis there typically are small raised smooth painless sores in the genital area. The lesions are evident in a man because they are external but they may go unnoticed in a woman because they are internal and painless. Sores may appear on the tongue, lips, breasts, and rectum as well. Although these sores heal even without treatment, the infection persists and spreads to the rest of the body. The second stage of syphilis begins two to six weeks after the initial sores have healed with fever, joint pain, skin rash, and malaise. The infected person may then go through another symptom free period during which the bacteria spreads into the blood stream causing the third stage of syphilis with severe nerve and brain damage and heart disease.

Viral infections cannot be cured, but many can be controlled. Genital warts are very common STDs caused by the Human Papilloma Virus (HPV). The warts may be flat or raised. They may be pink, white, or brown. They appear on the genitals or in the perianal region. They are painless and may occur in clusters. Nearly every sexually active person will have HPV at some point. It is the most common sexually-transmitted infection in the U.S. More than 40 types of HPV can be spread sexually. You can get them through vaginal, anal, or oral sex. Genital warts have been associated with cancer of the cervix, penis and mouth. Three vaccines (Cevarix, Gardasil, Gardasil-9) protect against these cancers. Gardasil and Gardasil-9 also protect against genital warts, vaginal cancer, and anal cancer. The CDC recommends young women ages 11 to 26 and young men ages 11 to 21 get vaccinated for HPV. A Pap smear can show most cervical cancers caused by HPV early on. Possible treatments include freezing, surgical removal, or use of topical medications, depending on circumstances. As with many other viral infections, genital warts can recur. Both partners should be treated and a condom should be used during intercourse to reduce the risk of reinfection.

Genital herpes is an infection caused by the herpes simplex virus (HSV). HSV1 usually causes cold sores and fever blisters around the mouth and HSV2 causes genital herpes. Either may cause infections in both the genitals and the mouth. Genital herpes is characterized by painful blisters in the genital area; however, this infection may also occur without symptoms. Herpes is always contagious and can be transmitted by direct skin to skin contact with the affected area even when there are no visible signs of infection. The disease is even more contagious when sores are present. Genital herpes may increase the risk of cervical cancer. Genital herpes is never permanently cured but can be controlled with oral medications.

Other viral sexually transmitted viral diseases which can have a major impact on your life include hepatitis B (HB), hepatitis C (HC), and HIV infection (Human Immunodeficiency Virus). Hepatitis B and C may be completely asymptomatic and may lead to permanent liver damage such as cirrhosis and liver cancer. The Hepatitis B and C viruses are mostly transmitted through exposure to infective blood. This may happen through transfusions of contaminated blood and blood products, contaminated injections during medical procedures, through injection drug use and also through semen, and other body fluids. While safe and effective vaccines are available to prevent HB, no vaccines have been developed against HC.

HIV causes acquired immunodeficiency syndrome (AIDS). HIV attacks the immune system, greatly lowering the ability to fight infections and cancer. An infected person may be asymptomatic for many years while the virus keeps on weakening the immune system. Young adults diagnosed with HIV infection contracted the virus during adolescence. The presence of HIV is detected by blood tests for the antibodies that the body produces to fight the infection. This test is widely available.

Awareness of HIV has increased over the last few decades, but it remains a prominent health issue worldwide. According to the World Health Organization

(WHO), about 1.2 million people died from HIV-related causes in 2014.

To help protect yourself, it's important to understand how the virus is spread. HIV is not transmitted through hugging, shaking hands, donating blood, or having a blood test.

HIV is only transmitted through bodily fluids, such as blood, vaginal secretions, semen and breast milk.

Direct blood transfusion is the route of exposure that poses the highest risk of infection. However, since 1985 all blood donors are tested for HIV. Even with these safety measures, there's still a small risk that HIV-infected blood may be used in transfusions.

HIV can also be spread through needle sharing, among IV drug users; accidental needle sticks in a healthcare setting; having sex with a person with HIV, both anally and vaginally. In particular, anal intercourse with a HIV positive partner is the sex act that's most likely to spread the virus.

It's critical to always protect yourself during sex, as using condoms is the best way to prevent the spread of HIV and other sexually transmitted infections. Remember though that even using condoms is not a complete, 100% guarantee of protection against STDs. The only certain way to prevent HIV and other STDs is to abstain from sexual intercourse.

HIV can also be transmitted to the fetus during pregnancy or to the baby through breastfeeding, as well as during delivery. If you get pregnant, it's important to be tested for HIV, among other diseases. If you are positive, anti-HIV drugs can be initiated, which will lower the risk of transmitting HIV to the baby during pregnancy and labor.

Although there is no cure for HIV or AIDS, many medications are now available that can slow the disease process in many people.

If you have been diagnosed with one sexually transmitted disease, it is a good idea to be tested for others because several STDs may actually occur together. If you notice redness or swelling in your genital area, open sores, blisters, discharge, local pain and irritation, consult your physician for further examination.

(https://aidsinfo.nih.gov/) (http://www.healthline.com/health/hiv-aids/hiv-transmission-rates)

Pregnancy and Prevention

Teenage pregnancy is defined as a teenage girl, usually within the ages of 13-19, becoming pregnant. The term in everyday speech usually refers to girls who have not reached legal adulthood, which varies across the world, who become pregnant.

Many adolescents are unaware of the risks associated with sexual intercourse. Besides STDs, the possibility of the teenage girl's becoming pregnant is all too real.

Factors that put teenage girls at risk for pregnancy include peer pressure to engage in sexual activity, use of alcohol and drugs, poverty, low self-esteem, exposure to abuse and violence, lack of education and information about reproductive sexual health and lack of access to tools that prevent pregnancies. Teen pregnancy and motherhood can have a negative socio- economic and psychological impact on the teen mother and her child. Pregnant teenagers, particularly those below fourteen years, may have more medical problems during and after pregnancy than older women. Pregnant teenage girls and teenage mothers are more likely to drop out of school, be unemployed, have no or low qualifications, live in poverty, suffer from depression and have low self-esteem.

Since unplanned teenage pregnancy is a widespread problem in our society, all adolescents should be counseled professionally about contraceptive methods. Many health professionals promote sexual abstinence as the best way to avoid teenage pregnancy and STDs.

STDs during pregnancy can have devastating effects on the fetus and newborn child. These diseases may affect one part of the infant's body such as the eyes, the brain, the lungs, the skin, or they may involve multiple organs. The infections in the newborn may manifest as conjunctivitis, pneumonia, encephalitis, meningitis, hepatitis, skin lesions, and can cause mental and growth retardation, and even early death. Syphilis, HIV, and hepatitis B are acquired by the fetus during pregnancy. Micro-organisms such as chlamydia, gonococcus and herpes are transmitted to the newborn during delivery by passage through an infected maternal genital tract. Regular prenatal care with screening for these diseases is therefore critical to the welfare of both mother and child. Prenatal care also involves counseling about the dangers of alcohol, tobacco and other drug use to the mother and child.

https://www.unicef.org/

https://www.slideshare.net/islamicyaqeen/teenage-pregnancy-13574603

Urinary Tract Infections (UTI)

A healthy bladder is generally free of bacteria. Bacterial infections of the lower urinary tract occur when bacteria ascend through the urethra to the bladder where they multiply. About 5% of adolescent girls may develop a UTI. UTIs are less frequent in adolescent boys and raise concerns about the presence of an anatomic abnormality of the urinary tract. For this reason, when male adolescents are found to have such infections, they should consult a urologist for additional evaluation. A urologist is a doctor who specializes in diseases of the male and female urinary system and the male reproductive system. Some women tend to develop UTIs after sexual intercourse. Symptoms of a UTI include frequent urination with pain or a burning sensation; after urination, there may still be a sensation of bladder fullness. If left untreated a bladder infection may spread to the kidneys. The signs of a kidney infection include high fever, chills, malaise, and mid-back pain under the lower ribs. This type of infection can damage the kidney and be life threatening if left untreated. People who think they may have a UTI should see a doctor promptly. Treatment includes taking antibiotics, medications that kill bacteria or stop their growth, and drinking plenty of fluids. There are also over-the-counter medications that may reduce the symptoms of urinary frequency and burning. Any person who has frequent, recurring, or long-lasting UTIs should consult an urologist for further evaluation.

Testicular Pain

Testicular pain may be caused by local trauma, infection, tumor, and testicular torsion. Testicular torsion occurs when the testis turns on its cord. Symptoms include severe local pain, nausea, vomiting, and scrotal swelling. Immediate assessment is necessary to differentiate torsion from other conditions. Surgical intervention is necessary in cases of testicular torsion to avoid loss of the testicle. All cases of testicular pain need prompt medical evaluation and specific treatments as well. Many testicular cancers do not cause pain. It is, therefore, advisable for young men to begin a monthly self-examination in order to detect changes early.

Body Hair

A wide range of normal hair growth exists for women and men. This variation is largely based on ethnic predisposition. Caucasians generally have more hair than do Blacks, Asians, or Native Americans. Asians rarely have facial hair or body hair except in the axillary and pubic regions. White women of Mediterranean ancestry have more hair growth and a higher incidence of excess facial hair than do those of Nordic ancestry. Excessive hair growth in areas that are not usually hairy is generally a benign condition determined by familial background and ethnic heritage. This condition, termed hirsutism, may also be caused by a variety of medical conditions. Hypothyroidism causes an elevation in the testosterone level that may result in the growth of long, fine, soft, unpigmented hair. One of the most common causes of hirsutism in women is the polycystic ovary syndrome. People with anorexia nervosa and bulimia frequently develop fine, dark hair on the face, trunk, and arms which may be quite extensive. Certain drugs such as anabolic steroids may also cause hirsutism. If you are concerned that you have developed excessive body hair, a medical evaluation is warranted. Once an underlying medical condition is excluded, oral contraceptives may be one treatment option. Excess body hair can cause concern about one's appearance, but significant cosmetic improvement is now possible. Shaving is the simplest way to remove unwanted hair; while this does not cause an increase in the rate of hair growth, it may synchronize hair growth cycles, giving the appearance of increased growth. Commercially available hair bleach with hydrogen peroxide is also an inexpensive way of making facial hair less noticeable. Chemical depilatory creams are effective but frequently cause skin irritation when applied to the face. They may also seem messy and may have an offensive odor. Plucking can be useful when only a few hairs are present, such as the eyebrows and around the nipples, but may cause folliculitis and ingrown hairs. Waxing involves applying melted wax to the involved skin area. The wax is allowed to cool and is then stripped off, removing the hair imbedded in it. The result of waxing lasts two to six weeks which is longer than chemical depilatory creams because waxing removes the hair from the follicle below the surface of the skin. Electrolysis is the only effective method of permanent hair removal. While this process prevents subsequent growth from the hair follicle, it may take repeated procedures to achieve this result. This method is more costly, may be somewhat painful, and requires a well-trained professional to minimize possible complications such as scarring and post-inflammatory hyperpigmentation.

Musculoskeletal Problems

Physically active people often develop pain/discomfort in the muscles and joints. Cramps in the muscles are a common condition that occurs during or after exercise, especially in hot weather and without sufficient warm-up. Cramping makes the muscles feel like hard knots and is very painful. Dehydration with low electrolyte levels of sodium, potassium, and magnesium is often a triggering factor. To prevent cramps, drink plenty of fluids before and during exercise, allow sufficient time for warm-up, and stretch after the exercise to keep the muscles relaxed. Many sport injuries are due to overuse and can be avoided by proper conditioning and training. Over-use injuries include bursitis and tendinitis, such as tennis elbow, Achilles tendinitis which causes pain in the back of the heel, and patellar tendinitis which causes pain around the kneecap. A bursa is a small sac filled with fluid that allows the muscle to slide easily over other muscles or bones. Tendons are tough, rope-like fibers that connect the muscles to the bones. Over-use of a joint may cause inflammation of the bursa or tendon with resulting pain. Bursitis and tendinitis can occur at several different places in the body. They usually resolve in a few days to weeks if you avoid using the affected joint; anti-inflammatory pain medications such as ibuprofen or naproxen may help. Plantar fasciitis is a painful condition that occurs when the thick fibrous tissue at the bottom of the foot (plantar fascia) becomes inflamed. Athletes, especially runners and those who are overweight tend to develop plantar fasciitis. Trauma is another common cause of sports injuries leading to strains, sprains, dislocations, and fractures. A strain is an injury caused by over-stretching a muscle. A sprain is an injury to the muscles, ligaments, and tendons around a joint. A dislocation is the separation of two bones that form a joint. A fracture is a broken bone. Some pain and swelling occur with all these injuries. Most minor strains and sprains can be treated at home, but more severe problems need professional evaluation and care. The biggest challenge for most people with sports injuries is to rest enough to allow healing without losing overall conditioning. Activities that stress the injured area must be avoided. Swimming or biking will not worsen sore ankles or feet. Walking or biking will not aggravate sore shoulders or elbows. It is important not to rush a return to the activity that caused the injury. A few days of reduced activity or rest when you feel the first twinge of pain may help to avoid more serious problems.

Back pain can be caused by an injury to the bones and ligaments of the spine or by incorrect posture. The back includes the vertebral bodies (the bones of the spine), their joints, the discs that separate the vertebral bodies and absorb shock as you move, and the muscles and ligaments that hold it all together. You can sprain or strain ligaments or muscles from a sudden or improper movement or by overuse. Improper posture places too much stress on your back leading to discomfort and back pain. The more time spent sitting at desks, in cars, or in front of the TV, the more we must do to prevent back pain. This includes taking breaks from sedentary activity, using the abdominal muscles to counter strain on the back muscles, maintaining an ideal body weight to reduce the load on the lower back, and maintaining flexibility through regular stretching and exercise. Heavy back packs may cause back, neck and shoulder pain and possibly even problems with spinal development because of added strain on the musculoskeletal structures of the back.

Neck pain can be caused by injury to the bones and ligaments of the cervical spine, by incorrect posture, or by arthritis in older adults. The pain and stiffness result from a spasm of the muscles or from inflammation. Neck problems often cause headaches or pain in the shoulders, upper back, or down the arms. Most neck pain that is not due to arthritis or an injury is completely avoidable. Once again, good posture and exercise are important to prevent neck pain. Sleeping with the neck twisted, lying down in an awkward position to watch TV or read, sitting with the neck bent excessively, or sudden jerky movements of the head and neck (whiplash), or a direct blow to the neck may cause significant muscle spasm resulting in neck pain.

Other medical conditions beside injury and poor posture may cause musculosketal problems. Scoliosis is a back condition that should be screened for during adolescence. It is a lateral deviation of the spine with structural changes of the vertebral bodies. Sixty to eighty percent of cases occur in girls. Scoliosis may be suspected when one shoulder seems higher than the other, when one hip seems more prominent than the other or when clothes do not hang straight. An initial symptom may be the occurrence of fatigue in the lower back after prolonged sitting or standing which may later develop into backache. During the yearly physical examination from ages ten to fourteen, it is important for your doctor to examine your spine; this is best done when you bend forward because the spinal curve is more pronounced in this position. The greater the curve of the spine, the greater the likelihood of progression and worsening after skeletal maturity. To correct the problem and prevent deformity, a prompt referral to an orthopedist specialized in the treatment of scoliosis is highly recommended. Treatment options include wearing a brace or a cast or corrective surgery. Scoliosis and its treatment may threaten the teenager's self-image. Counseling and emotional support are a very important part of the care of teenagers with scoliosis.

Scheuermann's disease is a condition resulting in back pain and kyphosis (forward curvature of the spine) due to changes in the vertebral bodies, with resulting hunch back appearance. Scheuermann's disease is among the most frequent sources of back pain in young people, with pain more likely to follow either exertion or long periods of inactivity. The cause is unclear but local trauma may play a role. Typical symptoms include mild backache and a "round-shouldered" posture. It presents in adolescence with boys being more frequently affected. It is usually diagnosed during the routine medical examination. As in scoliosis, referral to a specialist is indicated. Treatment may be avoidance of strenuous activities and weight bearing on the spine, rest on a rigid mattress, use of a spinal brace or surgery.

Osgood-Schlatter disease is a common cause of knee pain in growing adolescents. It is an inflammation of the area just below the knee where the tendon from the kneecap (patellar tendon) attaches to the shinbone (tibia). Osgood-Schlatter disease most often occurs during growth spurts, when bones, muscles, tendons, and other structures are changing rapidly. Because physical activity puts additional stress on bones and muscles, children who participate in athletics — especially running and jumping sports - are at an increased risk for this condition. However, less active adolescents may also experience this problem.

In most cases of Osgood-Schlatter disease, simple measures like rest, over-the-counter medication, and stretching and strengthening exercises will relieve pain and allow a return to daily activities. The cause may be excessive traction by the patellar tendon on its bony insertion. The condition usually resolves spontaneously in a few weeks or months. Treatment consists of avoidance of sports and excessive exercise involving deep knee bending as well as the use of anti-inflammatory pain reliever. (https://bouldercentre.com/osgood-schlatter-disease-knee-pain/, http://orthoinfo.aaos.org).

Another cause for joints to become painful and swollen is a vast array of rheumatologic diseases. Often these conditions are associated with symptoms of fever, malaise or rash. Juvenile rheumatoid arthritis begins before sixteen years of age and may involve both large (hips, knees, ankles and elbows) and small (fingers and toes) joints. Rheumatic fever is a complex disease with arthritis of multiple joints that is a complication of streptococcal infection. A swollen and painful joint can also result from infection with bacteria and other infectious agents. Signs of infection such as fever and chills are usually present. If not promptly treated, the joint may be destroyed. Medical evaluation is required to establish a diagnosis and initiate appropriate treatment.

Genetic Diseases

Genetic diseases are a complicated spectrum of illnesses. You may think that they are something very foreign to your life, but some of these diseases are not uncommon, and you may actually have an affected relative, friend, or acquaintance.

Genetic diseases are caused by one or more abnormalities in the genome and are present from birth. The genome is the genetic material of an organism and is made up of approximately 35000 genes. A gene is a segment of DNA containing the genetic code used to synthesize a protein. A chromosome carries genetic information in the form of genes and contains hundreds to thousands of genes.

Genetic disorders may be passed down from the parents' genes or may be caused by new mutations or changes to the DNA. The science or laws of genetics govern the likelihood of inheriting any condition. There are some diseases that have a pattern of inheritance that has been well described. In some cases, the parents may each carry a gene for a condition that is not evident in them but may become evident in their children (recessive pattern of inheritance). In other cases, one affected parent will carry a gene that will be dominant over the gene from the other parent (dominant pattern of inheritance). Other genetic diseases are due to defects in the genes located on the X chromosome, one of the sex chromosomes. These diseases, such as hemophilia, affect males almost exclusively. Chromosomal abnormalities lead to genetic diseases as well.

The normal human karyotypes contain 22 pairs of autosomal chromosomes and one pair of sex chromosomes (allosomes). Normal karyotypes for females contain two X chromosomes and are denoted 46,XX; males have both an X and a Y chromosome denoted 46,XY. Any variation from the standard karyotype may lead to developmental abnormalities.

Neurofibromatosis

Neurofibromatosis, also known as von Recklinghausen's disease occurs in about one in 2600- 3,000 individuals of all races. This disease has an autosomal dominant transmission. That means, if one of your parents has the gene for this condition and the other does not, you may still inherit this condition. The severity of presentation may differ from individual to individual. Neurofibromatosis is characterized by pigmented skin lesions called cafe au lait spots, cutaneous and subcutaneous tumors called neurofibromas, and a variety of other manifestations which affect many different organ systems. One problem faced by people who inherit this condition is a cosmetic one. The tumors may be quite obvious and may occur in many visible areas of the body causing possible psychological consequences due to the insensitive remarks made by peers. This may lead to introversion and low self-esteem. In others, the lesions may cause significant medical problems. Tumors that develop in the brain can cause blindness, deafness, headache, balance problems, speech impediments and learning disabilities. Tumors that occur within the spinal cord may cause spinal cord compression or peripheral nerve compression leading to motor and sensory deficits. Another significant problem for adolescents with this condition is the development of skeletal anomalies, mainly deformities of the vertebral bodies causing scoliosis.

Cystic Fibrosis

Cystic fibrosis (CF) is an autosomal recessive disease: both parents must carry the genetic defect and the child must inherit both genes in order to have the condition. The parents are completely unaffected. This is considered the most common lethal inherited disease in the American Caucasian population with a frequency of one in 2,500 live births. In contrast, in the African-American population, it occurs in only one in 17,000 live births and one in 31,000 in the Asian American population. The presentation of this condition is probably more uniform than in the case of neurofibromatosis. Patients with CF have salty-tasting skin, frequent lung infections including pneumonia or bronchitis, persistent cough with phlegm production, wheezing, shortness of breath, poor growth, greasy, bulky stools or difficulty with bowel movements.

The patients have problems with their airways being colonized with bacteria early in life and becoming obstructed by the thick secretions that are produced. The other significant problem for these patients is a plugging of ducts in the pancreas that leads to problems absorbing food from the intestinal tract. In the past, patients with cystic fibrosis died around the time of adolescence or in their early twenties. There has, however, been a remarkable improvement in survival over the last thirty years. Patients now commonly live beyond their twenties due to the health care network focusing on a maintenance program to address their pulmonary and gastrointestinal problems.

Tourette's Syndrome (TS)

Tourette's Syndrome is part of a broader group of Tic Disorders, where genetic factors clearly play an important role, as these conditions are, in many cases, hereditary. A gene or set of genes that could be responsible for TS has not been identified yet. It is very likely that environmental factors and other unidentified factors may contribute to the development of these disorders.

Tourette and Tic Disorders are not as rare as they were thought to be. Research studies shows that, in the United States, about 0.6% of children between the ages of 5-17 has TS, affecting males more than females.

Symptoms manifest in childhood, initially with simple tics. Vocal tics are very common; they may begin as grunting or barking noises and evolve into compulsive, involuntary utterances.

Uncontrollable cursing (coprolalia) occurs in a large percentage of patients; this, as well as severe tics, may become physically and socially disabling. Drugs are used in an attempt to control the symptoms.

Sickle Cell Disease

Sickle cell disease affects about one in 365 African-American newborns (www.cdc.gov). It is an autosomal recessive disease that alters the main protein in the red blood cells called hemoglobin (hemoglobinopathy). A child who has inherited only one affected gene will have the trait, which manifests with minor abnormalities of the red blood cell count (mild anemia). If, however, the child inherits a gene from each parent, he/she has a much more serious problem. They will develop a significant anemia on their blood count. They have problems both from hemolysis, a condition in which the red blood cells are destroyed within the blood stream, and from vaso-occlusive events, which produce acute episodes of pain called sickle cell crises. Typically these episodes are characterized by bone and joint pain, chest pain and abdominal pain. They may be triggered by dehydration, infections and exposure to cold and may require hospitalization for evaluation and treatment. Sickle cell patients are also more susceptible to infections of the lungs or bones due to the inability of the spleen to perform the normal immune function. Routine health maintenance of these patients includes the yearly administration of the influenza vaccine and the periodic administration of the pneumococcal vaccine. In the United States, among patients with SCD, the median age at death was 42 years for males and 48 years for females.

Hemophilia

Hemophilia is a hereditary bleeding disorder due to deficiency of clotting factors. All races and ethnic groups can be affected by Hemophilia. There are two types of Hemophilia, Hemophilia A and Hemophilia B. Hemophilia A is four times as common as hemophilia B and is caused by factor VIII deficiency, whereas Hemophilia B is caused by factor IX deficiency. Some cases of Hemophilia are caused by a spontaneous mutation in the gene responsible for the production of the clotting factors, rather than being inherited from the parent.

Because the affected gene is located on the X sex chromosome, hemophilia affects males almost exclusively. Depending on the degree of deficiency in clotting factors, the bleeding episodes may range from mild to severe, and may be spontaneous or caused by trauma. In severe cases, mild trauma can cause extensive bleeding into tissues and joints, resulting in painful muscleskeletal complications. Patients with hemophilia should avoid aspirin and aspirin-like products. They also should not receive intramuscular injections, which may result in a large collection of blood in the muscle (hematoma). To prevent or treat the bleeding complications, fresh frozen plasma or plasma products that contain the needed clotting factors are administered. Prior to the routine screening for HIV, many hemophilia patients acquired the virus from transfusion of blood products. Detailed information about hemophilia care may be obtained from the National Hemophilia Foundation. (https://www.hemophilia.org/Bleeding-Disorders)

Down's Syndrome

Down's syndrome, also called Trisomy 21, occurs when there is an extra copy of the chromosome 21. It is not inherited in either an autosomal dominant or autosomal recessive manner, but results from a problem in the separation of the chromosomes. Babies with Down syndrome have an extra copy of chromosome 21, which alters the development of the brain and the body. About 0.7% of babies are born with Down syndrome, which makes it the most common chromosomal condition in the United States. Older maternal age affects the risk of having a baby with Down syndrome. A mother over 35 years of age may have an increased likelihood of having a child with this condition. However, most of children with this condition are born to mothers in whom age is not a factor, that is, whose age is less than 35 years. Children born with Down's syndrome may be recognized by distinct physical features. More significantly, they are prone to heart problems and may have a variable degree of mental retardation. There is a broad variation in the degree of physical and mental development problems among children with Down's syndrome. Therefore, some children with Down syndrome may be able to go to school, play sports and live a healthy life.

Conclusion:

What Does the Future Hold?

Rapid advances in medical technology have propelled the genetic code into a high profile arena, but, for most of us, the map of our chromosomes is unlikely to be available soon. Realistically, there is an easy and inexpensive way to anticipate the more likely medical conditions that may face each of us. Our closest biological relatives carry the genetic material from which our own genes are drawn. By looking at our relatives' physical and emotional traits and by inquiring into their medical history, we can see a pool of traits that we may have inherited, and take care of ourselves accordingly.

As we have discussed in earlier sections of the book, some of the most common illnesses in our western society are chronic diseases of the heart and blood vessels. Doctors refer to conditions that foster these diseases as cardiovascular risk factors: high blood pressure, hyperlipidemia (elevated cholesterol levels), diabetes mellitus, obesity, smoking, and a sedentary life style. Hypertension, diabetes and high cholesterol result from a complex interaction of several genes, as well as the influence of environmental factors, such as diet and activity level. These diseases are known as being multi-factorial in inheritance. If these conditions exist in close family members, it is wise for you to adjust your lifestyle accordingly. Many people nowadays follow a healthy lifestyle (low fat diet, exercise, smoking cessation or avoidance) even if they have no suspect family history, since prevention is considered to play such an important role in continued health.

This book is not intended to be an exhaustive review of medical diseases or an encyclopedia, but rather an overview of problems that are critical to teenagers and adolescents in this time of their life, a discussion of important behaviors that can affect their health now and in the future, and a framework on which to add new information.

In the book we have addressed preventive medical and behavioral issues of great importance in adolescence. Besides taking care of the more traditional medical problems as they occur, we believe that part of the challenge in keeping adolescents healthy now involves addressing different issues, such as alcohol and drug use, sexual activity, and violence. The increased mobility of adolescents makes them more likely to come into contact with new and risky experiences that may dramatically affect their lives and may even cause early death. We believe that educating teen's about the risks of certain behaviors can give them confidence in making wise decisions and bolster their self-esteem. Throughout the book we have addressed the risks related to drinking alcohol and driving, the severe health consequences of tobacco, drug use and unprotected sexual activity and the impact of our cultural stereotypes on self-image. We hope that the information provided will help you to become responsible for your own physical and emotional health. Invaluable on line resources and websites have been mentioned throughout the book. As these will provide you with a wealth of information on the particular disease process or topic you're interested in, they should not be a substitute for consultations with a health care professional, every time the need arises, and for annual checkups in the doctor's office.

Printed in the United States
By Bookmasters